AUTOIMMUNE PROTOCOL DIET

Dr. Wendy Sherman

© Copyright 2020 – Wendy Sherman - All rights reserved.

It is not legal to reproduce, duplicate, or transmit any part of this document in either electronic means or in printed format. Recording of this publication is strictly prohibited and any storage of this document is not allowed unless with written permission from the publisher except for the use of brief quotations in a book review.

Dedication

I thank my many friends and family members for their support and helpful suggestions: Kate, Rosy, Aly, Very, Dr. Rob.

I give thanks to God for the incredible energy, clarity, and support I received in bringing forth this book.

Table of Contents

Introduction **8**

STEP 1: UNDERSTANDING THE THYROID ANATOMY AND HOW HASHIMOTO'S DEVELOPS **11**

    Chapter One: Understanding Hashimoto's and Hypothyroidism 12
        The Thyroid Anatomy 12
        What Goes Wrong? 14
        Symptoms of Hashimoto's Disease 16
        Treatment and Management of Hashimoto's Disease 18
        Chapter Summary 19

STEP 2: UNDERSTAND THE AIP DIET AND HOW IT WORKS **21**

    Chapter Two: The Autoimmune Protocol (AIP) Diet 22
        What is the AIP Diet? 22
        How the AIP Diet Works 24
            Nutrient Density 24
            Gut Health 25
            Hormone Regulation 26
            Regulation of the Immune System 27
        How Long Should You Stay on the AIP Diet? 27
        Benefits of the AIP Diet 28
        Gut Restoration and Boosting of its Beneficial Bacteria 29
            Learn More About Your Body 29
        Identify Foods That Trigger Your Autoimmune Symptoms 30
            AIP is a Nutrient Dense Diet 30
            AIP Boosts Self-awareness 30
            AIP Boosts Contentment 31
            Grit 31
        Chapter Summary 31

Chapter Three: Beginning the AIP Diet..33
  AIP Diet Guidelines...35
    Gluten Free Diet..35
    Grain Free Diet 35
    Low-GI Diet..36
    Autoimmune Paleo Diet..36
    Nutrient Dense Diet 36
  Nutrients for Hashimoto's and Hypothyroidism..................36
    Vitamin D..36
    Selenium 37
    Vitamin A..37
    B Vitamins 37
    Vitamin E 38
    Iodine 38
    Iron..38
    Zinc 39
  The AIP Lifestyle..39
    Physical Activity...40
    Sleep Quality...41
  Manage Meal Times 41
    Stress Management 42
  Chapter Summary 42

STEP 3: MASTER THE AIP COMPLIANT FOODS, HERBS AND SPICES..43
  Chapter Four: The Foods Of AIP...44
  Acceptable Foods..44
  Foods to Avoid..45
  Basic Shopping List..45
    AIP Herbs and Spices (Fresh Or Dried) 45
    AIP Oils and Fats..46
    AIP Vinegars...46
    AIP Baking Flours 46
    AIP Sweeteners 47
    Other AIP Baking Goods..47

Other AIP Pantry List Items 47
Elimination Diet Guidelines 48
Reintroducing Foods 49
   Food Reintroduction Guidelines 51
   Suggested Food Reintroduction Order 52
   Food Reintroduction Journal 52
Chapter Summary 54
Chapter Five: AIP Meal Plan and Cheat Sheet 55
   14 Day AIP Diet Meal Plan 55
     Week 1 Meal Plan 55
   Week 1 Shopping List: 57
     Pantry Supplies 57
     Proteins 57
     Veggies 57
     Fruits 58
   Week 2 Meal Plan 59
   Week 2 Shopping List: 61
     Pantry Supplies 61
     Proteins 61
     Veggies 61
     Fruits 62
   AIP "Cheat" Sheet 62
STEP 4: LEARN DIFFERENT AIP QUICK MEALS 64
   Chapter Six: Great AIP Breakfasts 65
   Chapter Seven: Great AIP Lunches 105
   Chapter Eight: Great AIP Dinners 139
   Chapter Nine: Easy AIP Salad and Soup Recipes 182
     AIP Salad Recipes 182
     AIP Soup Recipes 197
   Chapter Ten: Easy AIP Desserts 224
   Chapter Eleven: Easy AIP Snacks 243

STEP 5: EMBRACE CONTINUOUS LEARNING ABOUT AIP DIET 259
    Chapter Twelve: Frequently Asked Questions 260
        Why the AIP Diet? 260
        What Does it Mean When an Autoimmune Disease is in Remission? 260
        How Do You Know Whether to Eliminate Foods for 30, 60, or 90 Days? 260
        Why is it Important to Wait 3 to 5 Days Between Food Reintroductions? 261
        Beyond AIP Diet, is There Something Else You Should Do? 261
        What is the Importance of Having a Shopping List? 261
        Is it Possible to Personalize Future Eating Habits? 262
        Ways to Save Money While on AIP Diet¶ 262
        What if You Do Not See an Improvement? 263
        Tips and Tricks for AIP Diet Success 263
Helpful Resources 264
Final Words 266
Resources 268

Introduction

Did you know that Hashimoto's disease affects about 10% of the entire USA population? Did you also know that 90% of people suffering from Hashimoto's are women, and 80% of hypothyroidism cases result from Hashimoto's? That is more than 35 million people suffering from Hashimoto's and hypothyroidism in the USA alone. These hard facts and statistics paint a clear picture of Hashimoto's disease and why people need to learn more about it.

Hashimoto's is an autoimmune condition that occurs when the immune system attacks and destroys the thyroid cells. This causes a swing between the hyper and hypo-thyroidism. The symptoms are attributed to the hypothalamus failing to produce enough thyroxine releasing hormone, which in turn impedes the release of thyroid stimulating hormones from the pituitary glands.

Hashimoto's is a genetic condition that is triggered by intestinal permeability and exposure to antigens; however, being genetically predisposed does not mean that a person will develop any symptoms or the condition itself.

Though the current medical position is that Hashimoto's is irreversible, research suggests that this may not be accurate. According to research, having a healthy diet, less stress and exercising reduces the chances of developing Hashimoto's and hypothyroidism. Some common foods that we consume daily such as grains, gluten, soy, corn, eggplant, peppers, potatoes, nuts and tomatoes can trigger Hashimoto's disease.

With the right dietary practices, the thyroid function can return to normal. This is because once the autoimmune attack ceases, the thyroid will heal and regenerate. During the healing and regeneration period, you must ensure the body receives all the micronutrients required for a healthy and functional thyroid.

This is where this book comes in handy! It contains over 100 Autoimmune Protocol (AIP) diet recipes that you can follow to ensure that your body receives sufficient amounts of the micronutrients that are required to ensure a healthy thyroid as well as ensure the thyroid heals and regenerates after a Hashimoto's disease attack.

Through a thyroid ultrasound and a thyroid releasing hormone test that determines the levels of triiodothyronine (T3) and thyroxine (T4), it is possible for your doctor to know whether the thyroid has healed. An increase in T3 and T4 indicates that your thyroid is healthy and your doctor may recommend gradual withdrawal and ultimately elimination of Hashimoto's hormone therapy medication.

The Hashimoto's AIP cookbook includes recipes and ideas to help you succeed in treating the condition with changes in diet and lifestyle. This book is packed full of delicious recipes and information to help you prepare to adjust and successfully manage your symptoms. You will enjoy good food and help your body stay healthy at the same time. You do not have to put up with boring and tasteless recipes in the name of a healthy diet. There are tasty yet healthy recipes that do wonders at alleviating Hashimoto's and hypothyroidism. Indulge in this book to learn about this and much more!

Dr. Wendy Sherman

STEP 1:
UNDERSTANDING THE THYROID ANATOMY AND HOW HASHIMOTO'S DEVELOPS

Chapter One: Understanding Hashimoto's and Hypothyroidism

To understand the importance of the Autoimmune Protocol (AIP) diet, you must first understand Hashimoto's and hypothyroidism. Hashimoto's disease occurs when your immune system works against itself by attacking the thyroid glands such that the immune system produces antibodies that attack your thyroid glands[1]. As previously mentioned, Hashimoto's is more prevalent in women than men, and it is the leading cause of hypothyroidism.

The Thyroid Anatomy

The thyroid is a butterfly shaped gland located at the front of the trachea and just below the voice box. Ever seen or worn a bowtie? The area it covers is where the thyroid is located.

The thyroid gland uses iodine from the food you consume to make two core thyroid hormones; triiodothyronine (T3) and thyroxine (T4) which it stores and releases to the body as required[2]. Most people barely know of its existence but the thyroid plays a major role in emitting the two hormones that regulate how the body uses energy. This means that the thyroid affects how energetic a person feels, how fast you burn calories as well as your heart rate.

When the thyroid gland is destroyed, it fails to produce enough thyroid hormones and as a result, it causes hypothyroidism. Hypo means lower than normal and signifies an underactive thyroid. When

---

[1] Chistiakov, Dimitry A. "Immunogenetics of Hashimoto's thyroiditis." *Journal of autoimmune diseases* 2, no. 1 (2005): 1.

[2] Liontiris, Michael I., and Elias E. Mazokopakis. "A concise review of Hashimoto thyroiditis (HT) and the importance of iodine, selenium, vitamin D and gluten on the autoimmunity and dietary management of HT patients. Points that need more investigation." *Hell J Nucl Med* 20, no. 1 (2017): 51-56.

the body lacks enough thyroid hormones, most body functions slow down and you may feel depressed, run down and experience weight gain due to poor metabolism.

The thyroid gland is made up of hundreds of tiny follicles that are responsible for creating the thyroid hormone. As aforementioned, the thyroid requires a substantial amount of iodine to function; therefore, there is a special pump that is tasked to move the iodine from the blood into the thyroid. The pump delivers iodine into the thyroid where it binds with thyroglobulin.

The thyroid gland works by combining the two core substances; iodine and thyroxine, that make up the thyroid hormone[3]. Thyroxine is an amino acid that is mainly derived from the protein we consume or manufacture in the body.

Note that the problem does not necessarily arise from lack of the two substances but a disruption in the assembly phase. The two substances undergo a series of processes that result in the attachment of four iodine atoms into one tyrosine molecule, referred to as T-4.

T-4 is one of the two core thyroid hormones that is examined in laboratories prior to declaration of a hypothyroidism diagnosis. T-3 is obtained once the T-4 loses one iodine atom. T-4 means four iodines are attached while T-3 means three iodines are attached. T-3 is the active hormone, while T-4 is less bioactive since it does not bind to the cell nucleus during circulation. Thyroid hormones are formed by stacking on iodine and vice versa. So, as hormones leave the thyroid

---

[3] Parvathaneni, Arvin, Daniel Fischman, and Pramil Cheriyath. "Hashimoto's thyroiditis." *A New Look at Hypothyroidism* (2012): 47.

gland, they pull off iodine atoms and gradually move from T-4 to T-3 to T-2 and T-1. This process is referred to as deiodination[4].

THYROID HORMONES

Credit: Designua /Shutterstock.com

What Goes Wrong?

The answer is genes. This is because one group of HLA genes triggers the thyroid to thicken or become goitrous, nodular or enlarged. Another HLA group of genes triggers the breaking down of the gland. As such, both HLA gene groups trigger structural changes. They are both responsible for the development of Hashimoto's disease[5]. This explains why a diagnostic ultrasound is always preferred during diagnosis. However, this does not mean that people with the gene will eventually develop Hashimoto's; however, if you are genetically

---

[4] Kong YC, Morris GP, Brown NK, Yan Y, Flynn JC, David CS. Autoimmune thyroiditis: a model uniquely suited to probe regulatory T cell function. J Autoimmun. 2009;33:239-246.

[5] Hiromatsu, Yuji, Hiroshi Satoh, and Nobuyuki Amino. "Hashimoto's thyroiditis: history and future outlook." *Hormones (Athens)* 12, no. 1 (2013): 12-8.

predisposed, you do not require a huge amount of environmental, health or diet stressors to trigger the condition.

Another thing that goes wrong is the immune deregulation that is triggered by numerous factors such as infections and low Vitamin D in the body. That said, for Hashimoto's to develop, three factors must be present; genetic predisposition, microbial infection and intestinal permeability/leaky gut.

In a nutshell, a lack of immune tolerance by the thyroid cells results in the production of antibodies that work against the thyroid tissue and end up destroying the thyroid gland. The initial inflammation that occurs as a result of Hashimoto's disease occurs when a genetically predisposed person is exposed to certain environmental and immunological factors[6].

Antigen presenting cells like macrophages and dendritic cells begin to invade the thyroid glands after the inflammatory changes present. Thyroglobulin; a main protein that is produced by the thyroid gland is also believed to be a major auto-antigen that plays a central role in Hashimoto's pathogenesis[7].

A major difficulty in accurate diagnosis of hypothyroidism is that most people with the disease tend to have normal TSH levels (Thyroid Stimulating Hormone). This is attributed to the fact that TSH is a pituitary hormone.

---

[6] Liontiris, Michael I., and Elias E. Mazokopakis. "A concise review of Hashimoto thyroiditis (HT) and the importance of iodine, selenium, vitamin D and gluten on the autoimmunity and dietary management of HT patients. Points that need more investigation." *Hell J Nucl Med* 20, no. 1 (2017): 51-56.

[7] Akamizu, Takashi, and Nobuyuki Amino. "Hashimoto's thyroiditis." In *Endotext [Internet]*. MDText. com, Inc., 2017.

Symptoms of Hashimoto's Disease

Most people with Hashimoto's disease do not portray any symptoms at first. This is because the disease progresses slowly. However, the thyroid gradually enlarges causing the front of the neck to appear swollen. The enlarged thyroid is known as goiter and may cause a feeling of fullness within the throat region[8]. Note that an enlarged thyroid is not painful and it may disappear after a number of years or upon damage to the thyroid area.

Hypothyroidism resulting from Hashimoto's disease is mainly subclinical, especially during its onset when it presents mild to no symptoms at all[9]. But, as hypothyroidism progresses, the following symptoms may present:

- Unexplained weight gain
- Muscle and joint pain, including reduced tolerance to exercises
- Memory loss
- Tiredness
- Trouble tolerating cold
- Thinning and drying of hair
- Constipation
- Depression
- Slowed heart rate
- Irregular or heavy menstrual periods
- Trouble getting pregnant

The thyroid hormone influences the function of body cells. The main function of the thyroid hormone is to boost the body's basal metabolic rate. Therefore, symptoms of Hashimoto's are as a result of

---

[8] Hiromatsu, Yuji, Hiroshi Satoh, and Nobuyuki Amino. "Hashimoto's thyroiditis: history and future outlook." *Hormones (Athens)* 12, no. 1 (2013): 12-8.

[9] Elte, J. W., Aart H. Mudde, and AC Nieuwenhuijzen Kruseman. "Subclinical thyroid disease." Postgraduate medical journal 72, no. 845 (1996): 141-146.

the decreased production of the thyroid hormone due to destruction of the thyroid tissue[10]. A decrease in the production of thyroid hormones affects the functionality of different body systems. For instance, when the cardiovascular system malfunctions, bradycardia may manifest, while delayed reflexes and slowed speeches signify a dysfunction of the nervous system.

Once the metabolic rate drops to critically low levels, a life-threatening condition referred to as myxedema may develop. It is characterized by severe bradycardia, hypothermia, altered sensorium and hypoglycemia. Note that development of myxedema can be triggered by stress, traumatic injuries, infections and surgery especially in patients with severe hypothyroidism. Tumors of the thyroid gland are also a symptom of Hashimoto's disease. The tumors can present as solitary or as multiple nodules. Additionally, the accumulation of matrix proteins like metalloproteases can cause swelling of the face and extremities. Though Hashimoto's is rare in children, it causes detrimental physical maturation and growth effects. It is believed to cause mental retardation and short stature in children.

Apart from the hypothyroidism symptoms, people with Hashimoto's disease may experience symptoms resulting from other autoimmune diseases. Such symptoms include rheumatic manifestations, confusion, fatigue and irritability. As a result, patients who present with symptoms like occasional irritability, confusion and depression are often misdiagnosed with psychiatric disorders since thyroid hormone deficiency is only noted once the condition has advanced and caused additional other symptoms as discussed above[11].

---

[10] Elte, J. W., Aart H. Mudde, and AC Nieuwenhuijzen Kruseman. "Subclinical thyroid disease." Postgraduate medical journal 72, no. 845 (1996): 141-146.

[11] Ajjan, Ramzi A., and Anthony P. Weetman. "The pathogenesis of Hashimoto's thyroiditis: further developments in our understanding." *Hormone and Metabolic Research* 47, no. 10 (2015): 702-710.

Treatment and Management of Hashimoto's Disease

Once Hashimoto's disease has been successfully diagnosed, it is managed using a thyroid hormone pill that a patient is required to take daily for the rest of their life. While taking the thyroid hormone pill, you are required to visit your doctor regularly to monitor the levels of the thyroid stimulating hormone in the body. Note that the thyroid hormone pill does not offer significant results immediately; you may have to take the pills for a number of months before the symptoms disappear[12]. The dosage is adjusted once the thyroid stimulating hormone levels change. This may especially occur during pregnancy, when taking menopausal hormone therapy, or if a patient develops heart conditions.

Being an autoimmune disease, the inflammatory symptoms that arise due to Hashimoto's disease can be successfully managed. This is done by following the right diet plan and ensuring that your body consumes sufficient micronutrients such as minerals, vitamins, amino acids and essential fatty acids (EFA). These are core elements that affect an individual's overall health. As a matter of fact, nutritional and medical science has attributed the onset of Hashimoto's and other health conditions to deficiency in one or more of the essential micronutrients.

This means that it is possible to manage and alleviate Hashimoto's symptoms by ensuring that you consume a balanced diet containing all the micronutrients essential to maintaining a healthy thyroid. The specific micronutrients that you should incorporate in the autoimmune diet protocol are discussed in this book with the aim of ensuring that you not only understand their nutrient value but also how they affect the thyroid hormones. This book focuses on helping people to recover

---

[12] Vaidya, Bijay, and Simon HS Pearce. "Management of hypothyroidism in adults." *BmJ* 337 (2008).

from Hashimoto's disease and hypothyroidism and ultimately lead normal lives.

Therefore, when you set out on the path to start the AIP diet, it's essential to understand that healing needs to be the number one priority in your life. You want to live your best life the best way that you can, and the way to do that is to make yourself healthy first. Ensure that you consume a nutrient rich diet and reduce your overall stress, including taking a less stressful position at work or reducing your working hours.

Chapter Summary

- Hashimoto's is the disease, and hypothyroidism is the primary symptom.
- Take action by reading far and wide about Hashimoto's and hypothyroidism because new information and management tips are discovered every day.
- Hashimoto's patients have three things in common: they are genetically predisposed to the condition; they have a leaky gut and microbial infections.
- The symptoms vary from one patient to another. Therefore, it is important to run the right lab tests and ensure that they are interpreted by a skilled medical practitioner.

STEP 2:
UNDERSTAND THE AIP DIET AND HOW IT WORKS

Chapter Two: The Autoimmune Protocol (AIP) Diet

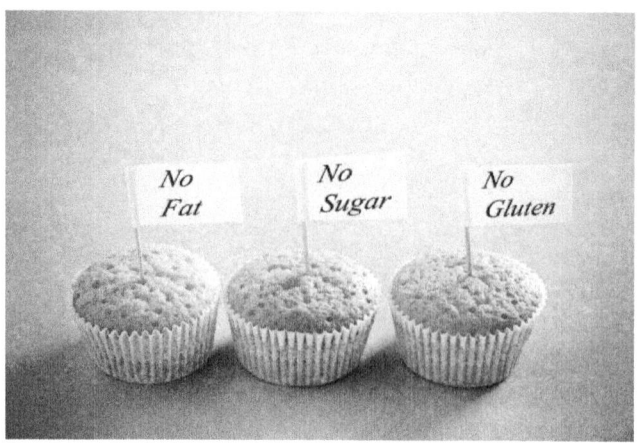

Credit: MShev/Shutterstock.com

What is the AIP Diet?

Despite medical management of symptoms using thyroid hormone replacement medication, people suffering from Hashimoto's thyroiditis continue to experience impaired quality of life and adverse symptoms. This is why the AIP diet comes in handy!

The AIP or Autoimmune Protocol diet is a science-based diet that advocates for a complete diet and lifestyle change in order to manage and ultimately send autoimmune diseases into remission. It is characterized by a lifestyle change that requires you to eliminate all inflammatory causing foods for deep gut healing of the leaky gut. Inflammation-causing foods are replaced with nutrient rich foods that address the body's hormonal imbalances and micronutrient deficiencies to restore the balance required for a healthy gut flora. Though it is recommended to follow the AIP diet religiously for 90 days, it reduces inflammation within 15 days as the body starts to heal gradually[13].

It is important to note that all chronic and autoimmune diseases are a result of a "leaky gut" and its immune response that triggers symptoms such as hypothyroidism. Therefore, by eliminating the inflammation causing foods, you eliminate the triggers that cause autoimmune symptoms and diseases. This ultimately allows your gut, body, mind and immune system to gently calm and heal itself naturally.

Years of immune damage resulting from consuming foods that are poor in essential nutrients and which cause inflammation causes a serious imbalance in our gut flora. This is what triggers a myriad of negative health effects that include poor nutrient absorption, fungus and yeast overgrowth in the gut, and prolonged infections and recovery times. The AIP diet focuses on restoring the body's microbiome; the healthy bacteria that keeps the body healthy. The diet encourages the consumption of high-quality probiotics mainly sourced from fermented foods because they are rich in healthy bacteria, bioavailable minerals and vitamins that the body requires.

The AIP diet is a special version of the Paleo diet that is characterized by a strict focus on nutrient density and the types of foods that should be eliminated completely. Some foods allowed on the Paleo diet are eliminated on the AIP diet because they contain compounds that can potentially harm the gut environment and stimulate the immune system to attack itself. They include nightshades like peppers and tomatoes, alcohol, seeds, nuts, and eggs[14]. Note that after some time, most of the eliminated foods that offer some

---

[13] Trescott, Mickey, and Angie Alt. *The Autoimmune Wellness Handbook: A DIY Guide to Living Well with Chronic Illness*. Rodale, 2016.

[14] Trescott, Mickey, and Angie Alt. The Autoimmune Wellness Handbook: A DIY Guide to Living Well with Chronic Illness. Rodale, 2016.

nutritional benefit to the body but have low quantities of detrimental compounds can be systematically reintroduced.

The Autoimmune Protocol is a lifestyle approach to the management of autoimmune diseases that focuses on providing the body with nutrient rich resources to regulate the immune system and trigger healing of body tissues while eliminating inflammatory stimuli. The AIP diet offers balanced and complete nutrition that discourages the consumption of refined foods, empty calories and processed foods. The AIP lifestyle on the other hand encourages stress management, sufficient rest periods and exercising for immune modulation.

How the AIP Diet Works

The AIP diet addresses four core areas that contribute greatly to the development of autoimmune diseases. As such, the AIP diet and lifestyle recommendations mainly target:

- nutrient density
- gut health
- hormone regulation
- regulation of the immune system[15]

Nutrient Density

The immune system requires a combination of minerals, antioxidants, vitamins, amino acids and essential fatty acids to operate optimally. As aforementioned, imbalances and deficiencies of micronutrients are the key contributors in the development of autoimmune diseases. Therefore, focusing on the consumption of nutrient rich foods triggers the synergistic micronutrients surplus to correct the imbalances and deficiencies with the aim of detoxifying the body system, regulating hormones and the immune system at large.

---

[15] Trescott, Mickey, and Angie Alt. *The Autoimmune Wellness Handbook: A DIY Guide to Living Well with Chronic Illness*. Rodale, 2016.

Nutrients also provide the body with the building blocks it requires to heal and regenerate damaged tissues.[16]

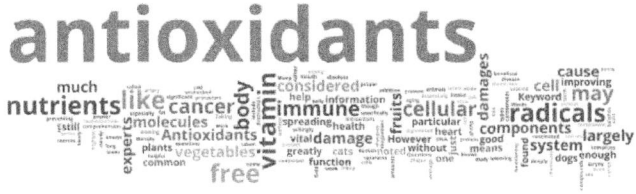

Credit: Pattagarn Temsakul /Shutterstock.com

A nutrient rich diet is made up of quality seafood, meats, fruits and vegetables. Some of the essential nutrients that are crucial at regulating the immune system and that most people are deficient in include zinc and Vitamins A and D. Note that fats are required in the body for the absorption of fat-soluble vitamins. Healthy fats are the mono-saturated and saturated fats. It is important to regulate consumption of saturated fats as well as to consume a balanced omega-3 and omega-6 polyunsaturated fatty acids ratio of either 1:1 or 4:1[17]. Note that a nutrient rich diet also boosts your stress resilience levels. This reduction of the effect stressors in your life may have a positive impact on your overall health and well-being by regulating crucial neurotransmitters and hormones.

Gut Health

For an autoimmune disease to develop, one must have a leaky gut. Leaky gut is an increased permeability of the intestine, which occur

---

[16] Soon, Tan Kar, and Poh Wei Ting. "Journal of Nutritional Disorders & Therapy."

[17] Marc Ryan, L. A. C. *The Hashimoto's Healing Diet: Anti-inflammatory Strategies for Losing Weight, Boosting Your Thyroid, and Getting Your Energy Back.* Hay House, Inc, 2018.

upon the loosening of the intestinal wall junctions. This allows undigested food particles, toxins and bacteria into your bloodstream.

How is this related to the food you consume? Some grain proteins known as agglutinins like wheat germ agglutinin and prolamins like gluten trigger intestinal permeability and encourage the overgrowth of harmful bacteria in the gut. Digestive enzyme inhibitors found in nuts, grains, dairy products and legumes cause gut inflammation, as does a high consumption of phytic acids. Saponins such as glycoalkaloids found in nightshade vegetables are also problematic to gut health.[18] Excessive consumption of alcohol and fructose not only increases the chances of intestinal permeability but also damages the liver. These are some of the foods the AIP diet eliminates with the aim of managing autoimmune diseases by boosting gut health.

To boost gut health and encourage healing, you should consume more vegetables, especially non-starchy vegetables because they feed the probiotic gut organisms. Foods rich in Vitamins K2, A and D, and the amino acids glycine and glutamine do a great job at restoring gut barrier functions. Above all, leading an active lifestyle and reducing stress levels also supports a healthy gut microbiome. The AIP diet recommended foods that enhance the growth of healthy varieties and levels of gut microorganisms.

Hormone Regulation

What, how much and when we eat affects a wide range of hormones that facilitate the immune system to operate optimally. For instance, eating too many sugars and small regular meals as opposed to eating large spaced meals destabilizes the hormones and stimulates the immune system. Hunger hormones are linked to stimulation of the immune system. Hence, minimizing snacking and eating large,

---

[18] Barrington, Kate. *The Hashimoto's Thyroiditis Healing Diet: A Complete Program for Eating Smart, Reversing Symptoms and Feeling Great.* Ulysses Press, 2016.

balanced meals is the best way of regulating hunger hormones. Note that intermittent fasting and skipping meals can cause cortisol levels to rise. The AIP diet is designed to regulate hormones and ultimately the entire immune system. The AIP lifestyle as a whole encourages the consumption of certain foods, getting enough rest, engaging in more physical activity and reduction of stress to regulate hormones.

Regulation of the Immune System

By now, you must understand that the only way to regulate the immune system is by restoring a healthy level and diversity of gut microorganisms. This is done by offering the body substantial amounts of micronutrients and hormones that support a healthy and strong immune system.

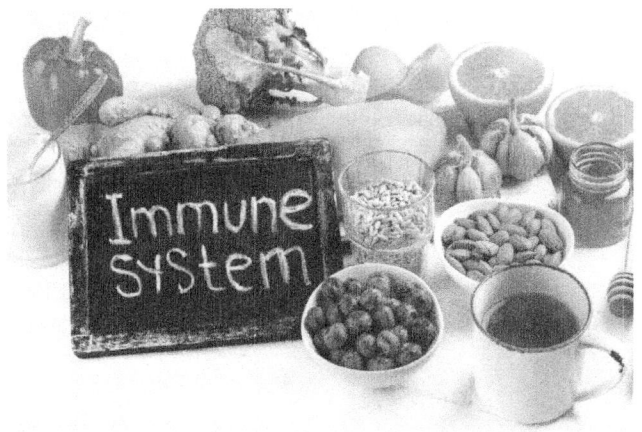

Credit: bitt24/Shutterstock.com

How Long Should You Stay on the AIP Diet?

It is recommended to follow the AIP diet strictly for a minimum of 90 days. Note that the AIP diet must be followed to the letter; any form of cheating can cause setbacks in your autoimmune disease remission and healing. Occasional cheating derails progress by triggering inflammatory immune responses that in turn cause a flare up of symptoms like hypothyroidism for people with Hashimoto's disease. The body will then require more time to recover from symptom flare ups, and that would mean more time for you to abide by the elimination phase protocol. For people who follow the AIP diet faithfully, it is possible to notice significant changes and reduction of symptoms within just 15 days.[19]

After the recommended 90 days, you can start reintroducing some of the eliminated foods, but this is done gradually. You will reintroduce the foods one at a time so that you are able to observe how your body reacts to the particular food. There are times when a person reacts to foods immediately after reintroducing them. In such a case, it is advisable to eliminate the food from your diet completely. Other times, it may be a sign that the body is not ready for that particular food and requires more time to heal and regenerate before taking in that food. It is important to understand that the reintroduction of eliminated foods should be a slow, gradual process that should not be rushed even if you are craving certain foods.

Something worth noting is that if there was significant damage to the body's immune system, you are bound to take longer before noticing a significant improvement to your autoimmune disease symptoms. This is because the immune system must heal and regenerate before resuming its normal functionality.

Benefits of the AIP Diet

Typically, the main reason behind adopting an AIP diet is to eliminate foods that irritate the gut and consume foods rich in nutrients which tend to reduce inflammation in the body. Following the leaky gut theory, one can easily learn how the condition begins and how to avoid it before it triggers the development of autoimmune diseases like Hashimoto's thyroiditis. The leaky gut theory states that there is a bacterial composition problem which arises in the gut thus triggering environmental inflammations such as viruses and toxins which breach

---

[19] Trescott, Mickey, and Angie Alt. *The Autoimmune Wellness Handbook: A DIY Guide to Living Well with Chronic Illness*. Rodale, 2016.

the gut wall and access other parts of the body. If you follow the theory recommendations, including lifestyle and diet, it is possible to not only alleviate Hashimoto's disease symptoms but also to recover from it completely. By adhering to the AIP diet, you can enjoy the following benefits and many more.

Gut Restoration and Boosting of its Beneficial Bacteria

The AIP diet is a healing and restoration diet that aims at restoring gut health and integrity in order to alleviate inflammation symptoms. For people with autoimmune diseases like Hashimoto's, this has a big impact; improving quality of life and general body health. The leaky gut syndrome that triggers autoimmune disease symptoms like hypothyroidism is a condition characterized by the passing of bacteria and toxins through intestinal walls. This causes symptoms like food sensitivity, digestion issues and inflammation.[20] The AIP diet emphasizes the elimination of inflammation triggering foods to prevent leaky gut syndrome and restore gut health. Diet plays a major role in the formation and effectiveness of beneficial gut bacteria. AIP enhances the health of the gut microbiome, which plays a major role in ensuring general body health, weight control and body immunity.

Learn More About Your Body

The AIP diet is a total lifestyle change that helps you understand your body and why it behaves the way it does sometimes. You will learn how your diet affects your health, immune system and resilience to autoimmune diseases. Such information gives you the impetus you need to take good care of your body by adopting a long-term nutritious diet that is not only healthy but also tasty. You will consume foods that meet your nutritional needs and learn ways of making the foods

---

[20] Lemes, de Andrade Isadora, and M. S. Filippovich. "AUTOIMMUNE PROTOCOL: THE USE OF DIET AND LIFESTYLE TO REGULATE THE IMMUNE SYSTEM." pp. 404-406. 2019

interesting and tasty. Healthy food does not have to be boring and tasteless.

Identify Foods That Trigger Your Autoimmune Symptoms

The Autoimmune Protocol is a diet that eliminates the consumption of inflammation causing foods and then later reintroduces them once a patient has recorded significant improvement or remission of an autoimmune disease. Though following the diet may be challenging during the initial stages, identifying the foods that trigger your inflammatory symptoms is the first step towards healing and preventing a relapse of an autoimmune disease. Above all, you get to learn the best foods to consume at different times of the day and which of the nutrient dense foods enhance immunity.

AIP is a Nutrient Dense Diet

The AIP diet encourages the consumption of unprocessed, nutrient dense and anti-inflammatory foods like vegetables and foods rich in vitamins. This means that regardless of whether you have an autoimmune disease or not, you can benefit greatly from the AIP nutrient rich diet. Consumption of healthy and nutrient dense foods maximizes your health and prevents development of all kinds of chronic diseases.

AIP Boosts Self-awareness

It is almost impossible to achieve success with the AIP diet if you fail to check in with yourself consistently. Test things out to know what works for you and what does not because you cannot rely solely on external guidance. You need to rely partially on what your body tells you. With an AIP diet, what works for another person may not work for you. Therefore, you have to be your own master and guide; check food labels, cleaning and personal care products to figure out what is ideal for you. AIP is a puzzle that is unique to everyone; hence, a positive attitude and curiosity to learn are key to ensuring the success of your AIP diet at alleviating autoimmune diseases.

AIP Boosts Contentment

Though the AIP is mainly focused on foods and diet, health and wellness is not derived from food alone. There are other factors such as chronic stress, lack of physical activity, draining jobs, and negativity that also determine a person's health and wellness. As you embark on the AIP diet, it is advisable to change your lifestyle as well. Exercise more and manage stress by setting achievable goals and improving your relationships. These are factors that eventually boost your happiness, health and immunity, which will help you to fight and manage autoimmune and chronic diseases.

Grit

Embracing and adhering to the AIP diet requires both mental and physical toughness. Rejecting the tasty summer cocktails or the freshly baked bread is not easy. However, when you are dedicated to honoring what your body needs, you will put in all the effort you require to remain on the right track. The AIP diet does not promise a quick fix, nor is it convenient. If anything, it is the opposite of everything the commercial food industry offers. This makes it a challenge because you have to constantly overlook the tempting foods advertised on your TV screen or cell phone, in malls and in restaurants. Adhering to the AIP diet and lifestyle is a choice you make because you are determined to heal and regenerate your immune system and the thyroid gland specifically for people with Hashimoto's disease. Having the grit to stick to the diet guidelines and enjoy the benefits no matter how long that takes is quite powerful and ultimately fulfilling.

Chapter Summary

- The Autoimmune Protocol (AIP) diet is an elimination diet that reduces the severity of symptoms in people with autoimmune and chronic diseases.

- The diet focuses on eliminating different food types that cause leaky gut and inflammation. The eliminated foods are later reintroduced gradually after the immune system has regenerated.
- The AIP diet is even stricter than the famous Paleo diet since it restricts many foods that are allowed on the Paleo diet such as dairy products, eggs, seeds, and nuts.
- Though the AIP diet has the potential to relieve autoimmune disease symptoms, it must be paired with a healthy lifestyle in order to achieve optimal results.

Chapter Three: Beginning the AIP Diet

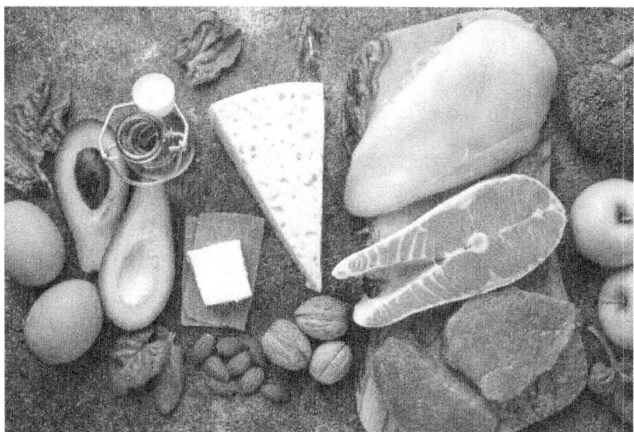

Credit: Yulia Furman /Shutterstock.com

As you embark on your Hashimoto's healing journey with the AIP diet, it is important to remember that there is no one size fits all diet plan. It is clear that the AIP diet alleviates and sends autoimmune diseases into remission by eliminating inflammatory causing foods. This does not necessarily mean that everyone reacts poorly to all the eliminated inflammatory causing foods. The diet eliminates all foods that are known to cause inflammatory symptoms among humans.[21] This explains the importance of the reintroduction phase where you are required to reintroduce one food at a time in order to evaluate your body's resilience to the food type.

Though the AIP diet has worked wonders for many people with Hashimoto's disease and hypothyroidism, it can be a difficult diet to implement. Many people suffering from autoimmune diseases know they can improve their symptoms through diet, but they do not know

---

[21] Lemes, de Andrade Isadora, and M. S. Filippovich. "AUTOIMMUNE PROTOCOL: THE USE OF DIET AND LIFESTYLE TO REGULATE THE IMMUNE SYSTEM." pp. 404-406. 2019.

how to get started on the AIP diet. Furthermore, if you have been consuming a regular American style diet all your life, adhering to such a strict diet protocol may be quite intimidating. Hence, it is advisable to take baby steps and begin by eliminating one food group at a time.

Note that for people who have lived off a dairy, processed foods and gluten diet all their lives, it is common to experience a short withdrawal/transition period before you will start feeling good on the AIP diet. In support of this statement, research indicates that casomorphins derived from a dairy protein known as casein and gliadorphin; a gluten protein found in wheat, are capable of binding the endorphin which is the feel-good receptor in the body. It is likened to the addictive morphine found in drugs. In light of this, some people believe that these foods (dairy products and gluten) are as addictive as hard drugs like heroin that bind the endorphin receptors.

Though some dieting and nutrition experts have dismissed this as exaggeration, some people experience withdrawal-like symptoms once they eliminate sugars, gluten and dairy products from their diet. The symptoms include cravings, headaches, brain fog and irritability among others. The good news is that once the body gets accustomed to the new and highly nutritious diet, you are bound to start feeling better and above all, healthier. You can expect to experience the results within 15 days and it gets better as the days go by. If by any chance you fail to experience significant results within 30 days, it is recommended to eliminate all meats and use fish as your main source of protein.

The AIP diet process allows you to be and feel more in touch with yourself by knowing what does and does not work for your body. Everyone has varying diet motivations, challenges and needs. Therefore, you should start by embracing your individuality and listening to your body. In the long run, you will have a lasting solution to your autoimmune disease and enjoy improved health.

AIP Diet Guidelines

Though no specific AIP diet plan is proven to be perfect for every Hashimoto's patient, there are a number of diets that have helped people with Hashimoto's disease to not only alleviate the symptoms but achieve full recovery. They include:

- Gluten free diets
- Grain free diets
- Low GI diet
- Autoimmune Paleo or Paleo diet
- Nutrient dense diet

Gluten Free Diet

Most Hashimoto's disease patients are sensitive to gluten. This means that gluten causes inflammation that is characterized by symptoms like cramping, constipation, nausea, bloating, fatigue, reflux, diarrhea, brain fog and gas. All these are factors that determine how good, productive and energetic you feel. A gluten free diet eliminates all foods that contain rye, barley and wheat among other grains. In the standard American diet, gluten is found in baked goods, bread, pasta, cereals and beer. A gluten free diet focuses on the consumption of natural, gluten free foods like beans, vegetables, eggs, lean meats, fruits, legumes, seafood, and nuts.

Grain Free Diet

A grain free diet is quite similar to the gluten free diet discussed above; however, a grain free diet focuses mainly on eliminating grains such as teff, buckwheat, millet, oats, amaranth, and quinoa. However, once you decide to settle for a grain free diet, ensure that you find other great sources of nutrients and fibers like selenium that are crucial for the recovery of people with Hashimoto's disease.

Low-GI Diet

This is also referred to as the low glycemic index (GI) diet. This diet is based on the index used to determine how different foods affect your level of blood sugar. Most people with diabetes type 2 rely on this diet to determine which foods work for them and the ones that do not. The diet is known to aid weight loss and lower the chances of developing heart conditions.

Autoimmune Paleo Diet

The Paleo diet simulates the feeding patterns of our earliest ancestors by emphasizing the consumption of whole foods that are not processed. The Paleo diet omits refined sugar, grains, refined oils, lentils, beans, potatoes and dairy. It encourages eating seafood, healthy fats, seeds, vegetables and nuts. On the other hand, the Autoimmune Paleo diet eliminates all foods that trigger inflammation and compromises the gut and is based on the paleo principals, but omits seeds, nuts, eggs and nightshades like peppers and tomatoes.

Nutrient Dense Diet

A nutrient dense diet emphasizes eating whole foods and a colorful combination of vegetables, fruits, lean proteins, fibrous carbohydrates and healthy fats. Foods under these categories include greens, fatty fish, carrots, beets, broccoli, berries, bananas, walnuts, avocadoes, legumes, and beans. It also encourages the use of anti-inflammatory herbs and spices like garlic, ginger, and turmeric.

Nutrients for Hashimoto's and Hypothyroidism:

Vitamin D

A number of studies have ascertained that there is a link between Hashimoto's and Vitamin D in the body. Over 80% of people with Hashimoto's were found to have low Vitamin D levels. As such, anyone with Hashimoto's should test for Vitamin D levels and seek to acquire it through sun exposure, foods or supplements. It is recommended to have 5 to 30 minutes of sun exposure on the legs, arms, back and face without using sunscreen. Where consistent sun exposure is not possible, such as for working adults who spend most of their time in offices, it is advisable to take supplements and eat foods that are high in Vitamin D like mushrooms, salmon, cod liver oil, tuna, fortified milk, sardines, and swordfish.[22]

Selenium

Selenium is a mineral that boosts immunity, fertility and brain function. The thyroid glands contain the highest amount of selenium in the body. This means that inadequate selenium levels in the body may cause thyroid dysfunction. Selenium can be obtained through consuming foods such as liver, eggs, Brazil nuts, halibut, sunflower seeds, oyster and grass-fed beef.

Vitamin A

Vitamin A works as an antioxidant that combats free radical cell damage that is associated with the development of autoimmune conditions such as Hashimoto's and hypothyroidism. The hydrogen peroxidase that is released when iodine is processed by the thyroid can trigger damage. As such, vitamin A regulates thyroid hormone metabolism to ensure that the thyroid functions optimally. Natural sources of vitamin A include sweet potatoes, carrots, liver, cod liver oil, winter squash, egg yolk, and whole milk.

B Vitamins

Most Hashimoto's patients have low levels of B vitamins as a result of malabsorption problems. For instance, you need vitamin B1 for stomach acid to be released properly. Hashimoto's patients have low stomach acid that in turn causes heartburns and indigestion problems. Low stomach acidity also inhibits the absorption of vitamin B12 that is obtained from foods of animal origin. For B12 to be

---

[22] Kawicka, Anna, and Bożena Regulska-Ilow. "Metabolic disorders and nutritional status in autoimmune thyroid diseases." *Advances in Hygiene & Experimental Medicine/Postepy Higieny i Medycyny Doswiadczalnej* 69 (2015).

obtained from food, hydrochloric acid and protease enzyme activities have to occur effectively in the stomach. This is why Hashimoto's patients, people with low stomach acidity and vegetarians are encouraged to take B12 supplements because they enter the body system in a free form state that does not rely on stomach activities for absorption. Sources of B12 vitamins include fish and red meats.

Vitamin E

Vitamin E and selenium work synergistically. Vitamin E acts as an antioxidant whose duty is to combat free radical cell damages. It is also effective at improving inflammation associated with Hashimoto's and hypothyroidism. Good sources of vitamin E include leafy greens, fish, and avocados.

Iodine

Though hypothyroidism is characterized by a lack of iodine, excess iodine is also harmful for Hashimoto's. Excess iodine increases thyroid peroxidase, which in turn triggers oxidative damage in the thyroid glands. Selenium supplements mitigate such excess iodine effects by playing the antioxidant role. However, where a patient has iodine deficiency, supplemental iodine is recommended to improve hypothyroidism symptoms. Great sources of iodine include sea vegetables, fish and shellfish.[23]

Iron

As mentioned previously, hypothyroidism is characterized by low stomach acidity which causes iron malabsorption and hence, low iron levels in the body. Low iron levels can lead to anemia, whose symptoms are similar to those of hypothyroidism like depression, weakness, brain fog, and hair loss. Moreover, iron deficiency inhibits

---

[23] Kawicka, Anna, and Bożena Regulska-Ilow. "Metabolic disorders and nutritional status in autoimmune thyroid diseases." *Advances in Hygiene & Experimental Medicine/Postepy Higieny i Medycyny Doswiadczalnej* 69 (2015).

the conversion of T4 thyroid hormones to T3. Iron can be derived from leafy greens, red meat, and liver.

Zinc

Just like other micronutrients, zinc absorption is inhibited by low stomach acid production. Just like iron, zinc deficiency inhibits the conversion of T4 thyroid hormones to T3. However, in cases where a patient records both low iron and zinc levels, concurrent consumption of the supplements is not recommended because zinc absorption may be inhibited. Note that supplemental zinc is said to be more effective at managing hypothyroidism. Food sources of zinc are fish, poultry, and red meats.

The AIP Lifestyle

Though often underestimated, lifestyle factors are crucial at managing autoimmune diseases and chronic conditions. The quality of sleep you get, stress, and physical activity all play a critical role at helping the body heal and remain healthy. Unfortunately, the current fast paced American culture leaves little to no time for self-care. You may understand the need for self-care, body and mind rejuvenation, but you end up prioritizing other tasks due to time factors.

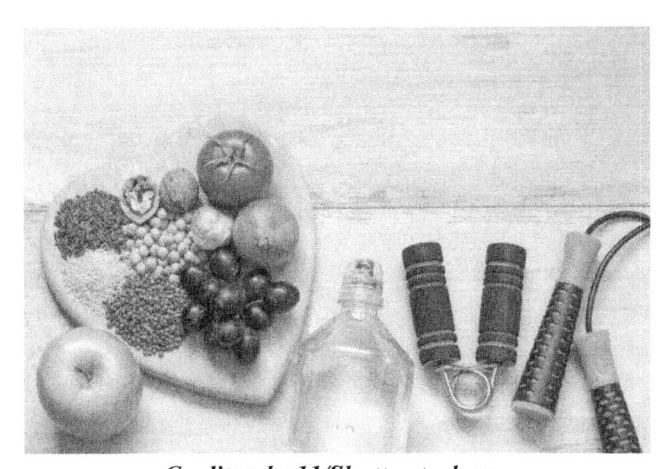

Credit: udra11/Shutterstock.com

Stress not only affects your health, but also your productivity at work and at home. There are different ways of dealing with and managing stress in your life. The stress management technique you choose is determined by the amount of time you are willing to spend as well as the cause of your stress. For instance, there are people who spare a few minutes each day to de-stress and refocus. Some people listen to motivational speakers, read books, listen to music or books, or share stressful issues with close family and friends with the aim of getting assistance or guidance.

Mindfulness meditation exercises are ideal for stress management. People who struggle with excess stress and anxiety are advised to seek professional help. Note also that having a negative attitude affects your quality of life and well-being. Hence, it is important to always focus on the good things life offers.

Adjust your daily routine gradually to achieve the AIP lifestyle so that you do not feel overwhelmed by many dietary and routine changes at once. There are numerous lifestyle factors that bar you from living a healthy lifestyle. Some of them are discussed below.

Physical Activity

Let's face it, not everyone feels the same about physical activity and exercise. Some people hate physical activities. Others struggle to find time to exercise and yet others love it! You must be willing to go the extra mile in order to manage and ultimately heal autoimmune diseases. Therefore, find a way to love physical activity! Start your physical activity by doing what you love or what is convenient for you. For instance, if you love swimming, having a good swim at least three times per week would not only be fun for you but also a way of keeping your body fit and healthy. On the other hand, if you cannot spare enough time to enjoy a good swim, you can opt to walk more. Park your car a few blocks away and walk to work or use the stairs instead of the elevator. If you have exercise equipment at home, use it while watching a show you like, or listen to a book or music that will distract your mind while you exercise your body. Limited mobility can be an issue for people with autoimmune diseases like Hashimoto's, so do what is comfortable for you and work your way up to more vigorous exercise.

Sleep Quality

A regular sleep pattern is important for maintaining circadian rhythms. Having regular sleeping and waking times helps to stop the hangover feeling you get as a result of broken or inconsistent sleep. If possible, have a calming ritual to unwind in the evening after a long day at work. It could be something simple like taking a candle lit bath and using your favorite essential oils, reading a good book or watching a movie.

Make your bedroom a haven where you find peace, rejuvenation and calmness. There should be no electronics in your bedroom and it should be very dark but comfortable when lights are off. Have optimal going to bed and waking times to ensure that you get enough hours of restful sleep. Also, avoid having dinner late, or at odd hours as it impacts the sleep cycle.

Manage Meal Times

Apart from prioritizing nutrient rich foods, it is important to have set meal times that you adhere to strictly. Take time to prepare some nourishing AIP allowed foods, then sit, relax, and enjoy the meal slowly. The current American culture often treats cooking as an extra chore that can be avoided by buying canned, prepared or fast foods that are omitted under the AIP diet plan. Therefore, you should start by changing your perspective about cooking. View cooking as a reward to yourself and a way of ensuring that you consume the right nutrients required to heal the body. Have 2-3 large and proper meals each day.

Since autoimmune diseases are often characterized by fatigue and pain in some cases, it might be ideal to adopt batch cooking where you prepare a week's food on the weekend, or when you find the time to, or when you are feeling strong. This is a time and energy saving technique that allows you to monitor what you eat and stay on track with your AIP diet commitment.

Stress Management

Stress management starts with identifying factors that trigger the stress in your life. Make a list of stressors and come up with ways of dealing with each effectively. Be kind to yourself by setting realistic and achievable goals to avoid causing unnecessary pressure. Set aside time to communicate with loved ones every day and involve them in your plans.

Chapter Summary

- AIP is an elimination diet that omits inflammation causing foods and then reintroduces them slowly.
- Nutrients are essential for the management and healing of autoimmune diseases.
- AIP diet is more effective when combined with AIP lifestyle that emphasizes stress management, quality sleep, and physical activities.

STEP 3:
MASTER THE AIP COMPLIANT FOODS, HERBS AND SPICES

Chapter Four: The Foods Of AIP

So far, we have discussed what the AIP is and how to begin implementing the AIP into your life through diet and lifestyle changes. I'm sure it seems a little overwhelming, and that is a natural response when starting a diet and making changes in a lifestyle, but now is where we get to the fun part. In this chapter, we are going to discuss some of the specific foods that are acceptable in the AIP, and we will also discuss foods that should not be consumed when following the AIP. I've also included food lists and essential shopping lists that you can take with you or store on your device. This will help you when you're shopping.

Acceptable Foods

Without further ado, let's get into the list of things that can be consumed when on the AIP diet. These items include:

- Meat and fish – it is better if they are fresh and not factory raised
- Vegetables – but not nightshades such as tomatoes, eggplants, peppers and potatoes
- Sweet potatoes
- Fruit – in small quantities
- Coconut milk
- Avocado olive and coconut oil
- Dairy-free fermented foods such as kombucha, kefir made with coconut milk, sauerkraut and kimchi
- Honey or maple syrup – used in small quantities
- Fresh non-seed herbs such as basil and oregano
- Green tea and non-seed herbal teas
- Bone broth
- Various kinds of vinegar such as apple cider and balsamic vinegar

Foods to Avoid

There is a list of foods that you are going to want to avoid consuming when you are on the AIP diet, as they may promote inflammation and cause unwanted side effects. Here is a list of foods you should avoid consuming:

- All grains such as oats, rice and wheat
- All dairy must be avoided
- Legumes such as beans and peanuts
- Nightshade vegetables such as tomatoes, eggplants, peppers and potatoes
- Sugars including sugar replacements (You can use honey and maple syrup instead)
- Butter and ghee
- Vegetable oil
- Food additives
- All forms of alcohol

Basic Shopping List

Here is a great shopping list that you can use to make sure that you are purchasing AIP compliant ingredients. Do not stray from the ingredients on the list because that will negate the protocol.

AIP Herbs and Spices (Fresh Or Dried)

Sea salt + flavored salt (e.g. lemon salt)
Cinnamon
Cloves
Garlic
Thyme
Parsley
Ginger
Basil
Bay leaves

Oregano
Rosemary
Mint
Turmeric
Dill
(Mace)
(Saffron)
(Lavender)
(Marjoram)
(Hibiscus)

AIP Oils and Fats

Coconut oil
Avocado oil
Extra-virgin olive oil
(Sustainable palm shortening)
(Tallow)
(Lard)
(Bacon fat)
(Duck Fat)

AIP Vinegars

Apple cider vinegar
Balsamic vinegar

AIP Baking Flours

Coconut flour
Tapioca flour
Arrowroot flour
(Cassava flour)
(Plantain flour)
(Tiger nut flour)

(Sweet potato flour)
(Water chestnut flour)
(Cricket flour)
(Pumpkin flour)

AIP Sweeteners

Raw Honey
Maple Syrup
Dried Fruits
Fresh Fruits

Other AIP Baking Goods

Beef gelatin
Baking soda
Shredded coconut or coconut flakes
Canned coconut milk
(Carob powder)

Other AIP Pantry List Items

Olives
Pickles
Fish sauce
Coconut aminos
Canned fish and seafood (packed in brine or olive oil)
Herbal tea (rooibos, mint, honeybush, chamomile)
Other teas (black, white, green)
Applesauce
Pumpkin puree
Dried seaweed
Lemon juice
(Sweet potato puree)
(Shirataki noodles)

(Kelp noodles)
(Chicory root "coffee")
(Horseradish)
(Real wasabi)
(Liquid smoke)

Elimination Diet Guidelines

As stated in the previous chapter, AIP is initially an elimination diet that omits inflammation causing foods that trigger symptoms of autoimmune diseases. The elimination portion of the diet helps people identify their food triggers and the particular symptoms of each food trigger. The elimination method is applied to determine specific food intolerances that a patient may be having.

When you regularly consume foods that your body is sensitive to, it is difficult to determine trigger foods and your reaction to each food. A good example is intolerance to dairy products. People who are intolerant to dairy products yet continue to consume them daily may experience symptoms like tiredness, bloating, congestion, acid reflux and joint pain. Unfortunately, they may not be in a position to pinpoint these symptoms as being attributed to dairy products. Every time you consume such foods, the body becomes less capable of protecting itself from the antigenic food. As a result, the symptoms will become more chronic and less specific because in the long-run, the body becomes sensitive to a wider range of foods.

Upon elimination of the irritating food for a number of weeks, you should feel better, more energetic and experience less acid reflux, less bloating and normal bowel movements. When you are reintroduced to the food after a number of weeks, the body will produce a more specific and stronger reaction that will help you to identify problematic foods and the reactions you need to watch out for in the future.

Common food sensitivity symptoms among different body systems include:

- **Respiratory system:** asthma symptoms, cough, congestion and postnasal drip
- **Gastrointestinal system:** burping, diarrhoea, bloating, cramping, constipation, gas, burning, acid reflux and nausea
- **Cardiovascular system:** palpitations, increased pulse rate
- **Skin:** itchiness, acne and eczema
- **Muscular system:** numbness, tingling, swelling, muscle pain, and joint pain
- **Mental:** insomnia, headache, brain fog, dizziness, depression, anxiety, and fatigue

During the elimination stage of the diet, you are required to eliminate the most problematic foods first and the less problematic foods last. On the other hand, during the reintroduction diet stage, you are required to start with the less problematic foods and end with the highly problematic foods.

Reintroducing Foods

One of the common questions among people starting the AIP diet is when they should begin the food reintroduction process. It is recommended to start food reintroduction once your autoimmune disease is fully in remission. On the other hand, if adhered to strictly, it is possible to have an autoimmune disease in remission within 30 days. Therefore, it is safe to start food reintroduction after 30 days if you followed the diet strictly. Alternatively, you can start the reintroduction process once your lab tests indicate a significant reduction of the autoimmune antibodies.

Note that it is common to have food reintroduction fears, especially if you have experienced a significant improvement of the autoimmune disease symptoms. You may be afraid that you will trigger the symptoms and have to grapple with their effects once again. This fear is normal and almost everyone who has gained relief upon adopting the AIP diet will have to face and overcome it! Though good for your body and health, sticking strictly to the AIP diet can limit your social life somewhat, because you may be afraid of eating out at restaurants or at other people's houses for fear of going off the AIP diet and triggering your symptoms.

To overcome this fear, communicate with others so they can support your food needs when you are with them. Understand what you can eat, and only eat that. Understand that it is important to gradually reintroduce some of the foods omitted under the AIP diet, so that you can determine the specific foods that irritate your system. Some of the foods that are initially excluded under the AIP diet guidelines are ultimately good for your gut microbiome. It is good to know what foods you will be able to have once you get the opportunity to reintroduce them into your diet.

Reintroduce one food at a time every 5 to 7 days. This allows you to have enough time to monitor your body's reaction to the food. Your decision on which food to reintroduce first is up to you, however, be wary of cravings!

Do not start the food reintroduction process if you are stressed, have an infection, have not had enough sleep, or have engaged in strenuous activities lately. All these are factors that could make the interpretation of a food reaction difficult. If at any point you are unable to determine which food caused a reaction, it is advisable to take longer between different food reintroductions. Moreover, you should limit consumption of reintroduced foods to small amounts and keep them well spaced apart if you want to achieve long-term results.

Some of the reintroduced foods such as gluten-free grains and alcohol should be occasional foods. These are foods that do not cause reactions when consumed in moderation but have the potential to undermine the immune system if consumed on a regular basis. Such foods are reintroduced to ensure comfort and flexibility during travels and when eating out.

Food Reintroduction Guidelines

Determine the food to reintroduce and be ready to eat it at least twice in one day. Then avoid consuming the food for 5 to 7 days as you observe your body's reaction to the food. Start by eating small quantities of the food and give yourself 15-minute breaks before consuming more. Should you experience any reactions during the 15 minutes breaks, stop eating the food. Once you are done with the first serving, wait for 2 to 3 hours before consuming your second and third servings of the food.

If you do not experience any symptoms during the 5 to 7 day wait period; it is safe to reincorporate the food in your diet.

Symptoms to watch out for during reintroduction:

- Symptoms that a diagnosed disease is worsening or relapsing
- Gastrointestinal problems like constipation, stomach ache, nausea, change in bowel movement frequency, bloating and heartburn among others
- Reduced energy or increased fatigue
- Increased or new cravings for caffeine, salt, sugar and fat
- Trouble sleeping, staying awake at night and feeling tired in the morning
- Headaches
- Mood swings
- Anxiety
- Pain in muscles, ligaments, and joints
- Skin changes such as pink bumps, dry hair, rashes, skin dryness, acne or dry nails

Suggested Food Reintroduction Order

There is no right or wrong way to choose your first foods to reintroduce. Some people will argue that the first food to reintroduce should be the foods you crave most; others believe that you should start with foods that are less capable of triggering symptoms or that have the highest nutrient density. The suggested food reintroduction process factors in the likelihood that a food will trigger a reaction and the nutrient density of the food. There are four food reintroduction stages.

The **first stage** represents foods that are less likely to cause reactions and are of high nutritional value. They include egg yolks, legume sprouts, legumes, peas, nuts or seed oil, seed-based spices and berries.

Stage two foods are foods that may not be well-tolerated and have a lesser nutritional value. They include chia seeds, butter from grass-fed cows, a cup of coffee daily, nuts, seeds, egg whites and alcohol in minimal quantities.

Stage three foods are foods that the body may not tolerate yet they have some nutritional value. They include; eggplants, sweet peppers, paprika, grass-fed dairy, lentils, and split peas.

Stage four foods are foods that may be totally intolerable and you may wish to never challenge them. They include tomatoes, white rice, regular consumption of alcohol, unpeeled potatoes, chili peppers, gluten-free grains and nightshade spices.

Food Reintroduction Journal

It is advisable to keep a detailed journal during the entire food reintroduction process. A journal helps you keep track of the food reintroduction dates, types of food reintroduced and the type of symptoms you experienced upon eating them. The journal ensures that you do not miss any subtle symptoms. Some symptoms may not show up within the 5 to 7 days waiting period, so keep a journal to track short- and long-term impacts of the foods you eat.

Design a food journal that works for you. Here is an example:

Date	Reintroduced Food	Symptoms
2/2/2020	Dairy	Stomach ache, joint pain
2/3/2020	Eggs	Bloating, gas

Chapter Summary

- Despite the common myth that the AIP diet is expensive compared to the popular American fast food diet, the starter AIP diet shopping list is basic and affordable. It incorporates most of the foods you are used to consuming daily.
- There are so many foods that you are used to eating that you can continue eating without concern. Meat and green leafy vegetables are very good for you.
- Some of the foods and spices that that must be eliminated include nightshades like peppers and also grains.
- The elimination portion of the diet helps to ensure that you consume only the most beneficial foods at the beginning of the AIP diet. This stage omits all inflammation causing foods with the aim of restoring the body's full and effective functionality.
- Food reintroduction should be done gradually to ensure that you do not miss important symptoms of food intolerance. This ensures that you reintroduce foods one at a time so that you clearly understand and can avoid future recurrence of the inflammatory symptoms.
- It is advisable to have a food reintroduction journal to help you keep track of what you are eating, and how it effects your body.

Chapter Five: AIP Meal Plan and Cheat Sheet

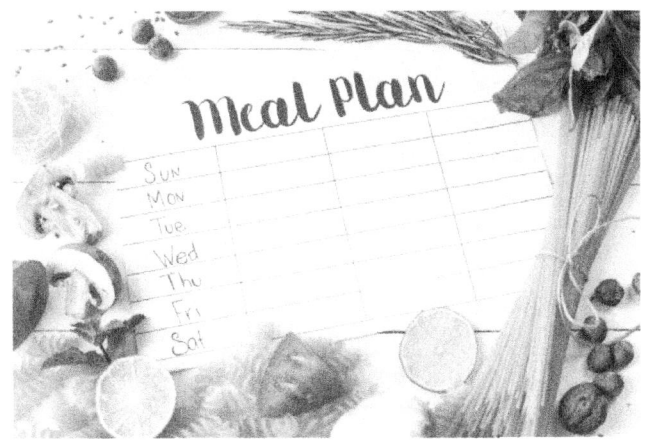

Credit: svitlini r/Shutterstock.com

14 Day AIP Diet Meal Plan

Week 1 Meal Plan

Monday

Breakfast: Chicken poppers and sausages with a fruit

Lunch: Beef bacon liver, avocado and cabbage salad with bone broth

Dinner: Stir fried ground beef

Tuesday

Breakfast: Classic AIP breakfast hash template

Lunch: Stir fried ground beef

Dinner: Chicken burger with spinach, sweet potato fries and avocado

Wednesday

Breakfast: Chicken poppers and sausages with a fruit

Lunch: Beef bacon liver, avocado and cabbage salad with bone broth

Dinner: Sweet potato fries with hamburger steak

Thursday

Breakfast: Classic AIP breakfast hash template

Lunch: Chicken burger with spinach, sweet potato fries and avocado

Dinner: Sweet potato fries with hamburger steak

Friday

Breakfast: Skillet Mexican breakfast

Lunch: Sweet potato fries with hamburger steak

Dinner: Chicken curry with turmeric

Saturday

Breakfast: Classic AIP breakfast hash template

Lunch: Chicken burger with spinach, sweet potato fries and avocado

Dinner: Plantain chips with tuna salad laced with avocado

Sunday

Breakfast: Skillet Mexican breakfast

Lunch: Chicken curry with turmeric

Dinner: Plantain chips with tuna salad laced with avocado

Week 1 Shopping List:

Pantry Supplies

- Arrowroot starch
- Apple cider vinegar
- Garlic powder
- Collagen
- Sage
- Turmeric
- Cinnamon
- Salt
- Coconut flour
- Beef broth
- Coconut aminos
- Shredded coconut
- Onion powder
- Coconut milk
- Avocado oil
- Coconut oil
- Olive oil

Proteins

- Ground chicken 3 lb
- Chicken breast 2 lb
- Ground beef 3 lb
- Tuna

Veggies

- 1 garlic bulb
- 1 butter lettuce
- Spinach
- Kale
- 2 zucchinis

- 1 cabbage
- Radishes
- Celery
- Onions
- Green onions
- Mushroom 1 container or small bag
- Cilantro
- Limes
- Shredded carrots
- Parsley
- Fresh ginger
- 5 sweet potatoes
- Purple cabbage

Fruits

- 4 avocados
- 3 apples
- Berries of your choice
- Any other fresh fruit of your choice, preferably fruits in season

Week 2 Meal Plan

Monday

Breakfast: Bacon, salmon and pesto salad

Lunch: Ginger salmon baked with fennel and beet salad

Dinner: Roasted pork chops with spring salad

Tuesday

Breakfast: Thyme-citrus turkey sausages

Lunch: Roasted pork chops with spring salad

Dinner: Sweet potato chili and carrot

Wednesday

Breakfast: Bacon, salmon and pesto salad

Lunch: Sweet potato chili and carrot

Dinner: Ginger salmon baked with fennel and beet salad

Thursday

Breakfast: Thyme-citrus turkey sausages

Lunch: Shredded chicken breast with chicken curry salad

Dinner: Sweet potato chili and carrot

Friday

Breakfast: Cauliflower oatmeal

Lunch: Ginger salmon baked with fennel and beet salad

Dinner: Shredded chicken breast with chicken curry salad

Saturday

Breakfast: Thyme-citrus turkey sausages

Lunch: Shredded chicken breast with chicken curry salad

Dinner: Beef liver with avocado and cabbage salad

Sunday

Breakfast: Cauliflower oatmeal

Lunch: Sardine salad

Dinner: Beef liver with avocado and cabbage salad

Week 2 Shopping List:

Pantry Supplies

- Ginger powder
- Garlic powder
- Sea salt
- Apple cider vinegar
- Coconut oil
- Turmeric
- Cinnamon
- Bay leaves
- Coconut vinegar

Proteins

- Grass fed ground beef 5 lbs
- Pastured ground pork 1 lb
- Pastured pork chops 2 lbs
- Grass fed beef liver 1 lb
- Pastured chicken breast 1 lb
- Grass fed beef roast 3 lbs
- Salmon 12 ounces
- AIP approved bacon 6 pieces
- Bones for broth preparation
- Ground turkey 1 lb
- Sardines

Veggies

- Carrots
- Cucumbers
- Parsnips
- 2 fennel bulbs
- 1 cabbage
- Oregano

- Thyme
- Sage
- Rosemary
- Mint
- Parsley
- Sweet potatoes
- Arugula 12 ounces
- Cauliflower rice

Fruits

- Avocados
- Grapefruits
- Lemons
- Oranges
- Fresh cilantro

AIP "Cheat" Sheet

The AIP diet is a strict, health-oriented diet that is a lifestyle especially for people with autoimmune diseases. These people embrace the AIP diet and later on adopt a Paleo diet version that works for them for life. AIP eliminates inflammation causing foods from your diet for a while, after which the foods are reintroduced gradually and in phases.

The AIP diet eliminates all processed foods. It also eliminates some of the foods that are often thought of as healthy but are linked to leaky gut and inflammation. These foods include seeds, nuts, dried fruits, nightshades, grains, coffee and legumes. The foods that remain include a few meats, vegetables and fruits that you should eat diligently for 3 to 8 weeks before reintroducing the eliminated foods. It is advisable to begin the reintroduction phase only once you are fully recovered from an autoimmune disease or when you feel fully ready.

Eliminating gluten can be difficult for people starting the AIP diet; however, they later realize during the reintroduction stage that their bodies cannot handle gluten. The AIP diet helps you discover the foods that disrupt your gut health and trigger the immune system.

For people who have been diagnosed with gluten allergies like celiac disease, everything they cook must be sterile; meaning that it should not have a touch of gluten. For such people, it is advisable to stick with vegetables, proteins and healthy fats.

Once you eliminate processed foods, coffee, seeds, eggs, grains and nuts, you may feel a bit lost during meal times because there will be no more "convenient" food options like bread, pizza, muffins and doughnuts among others. You must be ready to cook your own food to ensure that it is AIP diet compliant at every stage of preparation and cooking. As such, it is advisable to batch cook and refrigerate food. This way, you will have quick meals that are healthy and nutrient dense.

STEP 4:
LEARN DIFFERENT AIP QUICK MEALS

Chapter Six: Great AIP Breakfasts

Plum and Apple Cake

Macros:

Prep time: 20 minutes
Cook time: 30 minutes
Servings: 6
Fat: 5.3 g
Sodium: 12 mg
Carbohydrates: 48.5 g
Fiber: 7.2 g
Protein: 2.3 g
Sugars: 31.7 g
Potassium: 576 mg
Iron: 2 mg
Calcium: 86 mg
Calories: 228 per serving

What you need:

- ½ cup of arrowroot flour
- ¾ cup of coconut flour
- ½ teaspoon of baking powder
- a pinch of sea salt
- 5 ounces of prunes
- 2 red apples
- 15 ounces pumpkin puree
- ½ cup of coconut milk
- 2 teaspoons ground cinnamon
- 5 tablespoons of maple syrup
- ½ teaspoon of ginger powder
- 3 teaspoons of gelatin powder
- ½ cup of warm water
- coconut oil (to grease pan)
- baking dish preferably 11" x 7"

Steps:

1. Ensure the oven is preheated to 350°F and place the rack at the center. Grease your baking dish with coconut oil.
2. In a separate mixing bowl, mix arrowroot flour, coconut flour, sea salt, and baking powder. Set the mixture aside and allow it to rest.
3. Peel and dice the apples.
4. Chop the prunes.
5. In a separate and larger mixing bowl, mix coconut milk, cinnamon, pumpkin puree, apples, ginger, prunes, and maple syrup.
6. In a cup, mix gelatin powder with warm water. Stir until all the powder is dissolved.
7. Add the gelatin powder mixture to the pumpkin batter and mix.
8. Add all dry ingredients to the pumpkin batter and mix thoroughly with clean hands or a rubber spatula.
9. Pour the batter into the initially prepared baking dish and bake it for at least 30 minutes or until all the edges turn golden brown. Insert a toothpick at the center to determine if the cake is ready; if it comes out dry, your cake is ready!
10. Allow the cake to cool before slicing and serving it.
11. The plum and apple cake can be frozen for 4 months or refrigerated in an airtight container for 5 days.

Thyme and Rosemary Focaccia Bread

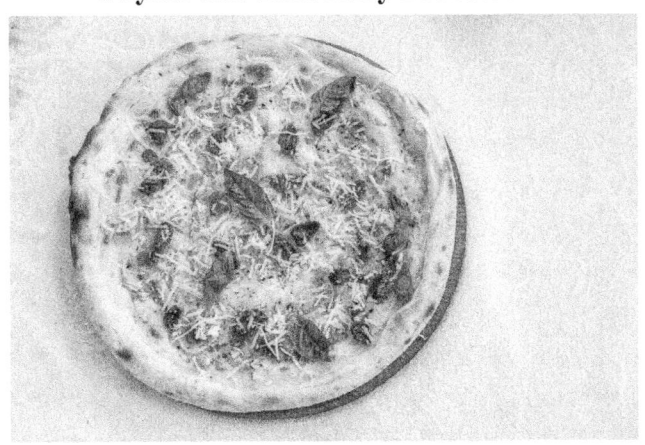

Credit: Morozov John /Shutterstock.com

Macros

Prep/cook time: 1 hour 50 minutes
Servings: 1 loaf
Fat: 26.4 g
Sodium: 954 mg
Carbohydrates: 45.5 g
Fiber: 3.7 g
Protein: 3.2 g
Vitamin C: 23.5 g
Potassium: 480 mg
Iron: 0.73 mg
Calcium: 55 mg
Calories: 424 per serving

What you need

- one cup warm water
- 1 tsp. maple syrup
- dry yeast 1 packet
- cassava flour 1 cup
- coconut flour ½ cup
- 3 tsp. dried rosemary for garnishing
- 2 tsp. dried thyme
- a pinch of sea salt
- ½ cup of melted palm shortening
- Baking dish

Steps:

1. Line the baking dish with parchment paper.
2. In a small bowl, mix maple syrup with warm water.
3. Once well mixed, add yeast and mix thoroughly. Give this mixture at least 5 minutes to start foaming. Note: the mixture must foam, otherwise it should be disposed of and the process redone. The foam lets you know that the yeast is working.
4. In a separate and larger bowl, mix the coconut flour, cassava flour, sea salt, thyme, and rosemary. Mix thoroughly using a rubber spatula and once done, form a well in the middle.
5. Pour palm shortening, yeast mixture and remaining warm water in the well in the middle. Use a spatula to mix all these ingredients until the dough becomes smooth and consistent.
6. Knead with your hands about 10 times and shape the dough into a ball.
7. Place the dough on the parchment lined baking dish and flatten it evenly using your hands. The loaf should be 1 inch thick.
8. Cover the dough with a clean, lightweight kitchen towel, place it in a warm place and allow it to rest and rise for 30 minutes.
9. Ensure the oven is preheated to 400ºF and the oven rack is in place.
10. Uncover the dough after 30 minutes and use a serrated knife to score it lightly three times at an angle.
11. Sprinkle some thyme and rosemary.
12. Place the bread in the heated oven and allow it to cook for at least 30 minutes or until the dough turns completely brown.
13. Allow the bread to cool completely before slicing and serving.
14. Keep it well-wrapped with a kitchen towel and store it in a cool and dry place for up to 5 days.

Green Smoothie Bowl

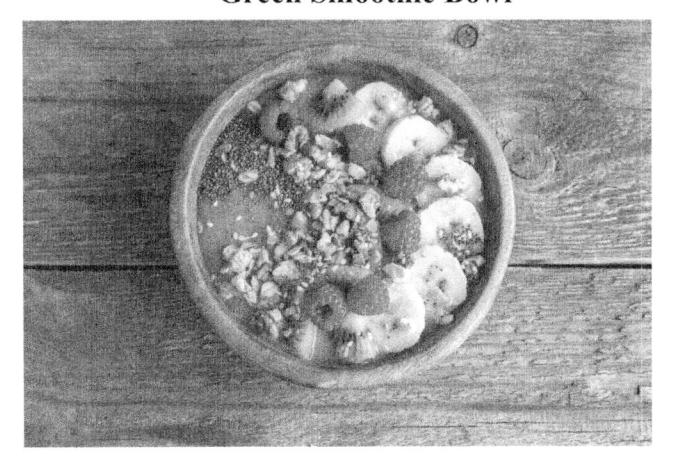

Credit: Oksana Mizina /Shutterstock.com

Macros

Prep and cook time: 10 minutes
Servings: 2 cups
Fat: 4 g
Sodium: 26 mg
Carbohydrates: 7.7 g
Fiber: 3.1 g
Protein: 1.7 g
Vitamin C: 41 mg
Potassium: 369 mg
Iron: 1.2 mg
Calcium: 40 mg
Calories: 64

What you need

- 2 cups of sliced spinach
- ¼ peeled and diced avocado
- 1 peeled and diced mango
- 3 big strawberries halved and hulled
- 1 lemon for juicing
- 1 orange for juicing
- 1 tbsp. collagen peptides
- fresh fruits for garnishing
- toasted coconut flakes

Steps:

1. Place the avocado, spinach, mango, lemon juice, orange juice, collagen peptides, and strawberries in a blender.
2. Blend the ingredients at high speed for about 30 seconds.
3. Transfer the mixture to a bowl and garnish with toasted coconut flakes, fresh fruits and nuts of your choice.

Cinnamon and Vanilla Granola

Macros

Prep and cook time: 13 minutes
Servings: 4 cups
Fat: 112 g
Sodium: 2770 mg
Fiber: 101.1 g
Protein: 40.8 g
Vitamin C: 2.8 g
Potassium: 1300 mg
Iron: 4.5 mg
Calcium: 65 mg
Calories: 1500

What you need

- unsweetened coconut flakes 2 cups
- tiger nuts 1 cup sliced
- coconut oil ¼ cup
- 1 tsp. vanilla powder or alcohol free vanilla flavoring
- Cinnamon 1 tsp.
- finely chopped apples ½ cup

Steps:

1. Preheat the oven to 350°F and put a rack about 6 inches below the broiler element.
2. Mix the coconut flakes, coconut oil, cinnamon, vanilla, and sliced tiger nuts in a large bowl.
3. Pour the mixture on the baking sheet, flatten the ingredients into an even layer and bake.
4. Stir the mixture a few times until the coconut flakes turn golden brown. This takes about 10 minutes.
5. Take it out of the oven, add the apples and mix thoroughly.
6. Let the granola cool and store it in an airtight dish.
7. Serve granola with fresh fruits and coconut milk.

Veggie and Protein Collagen Blend

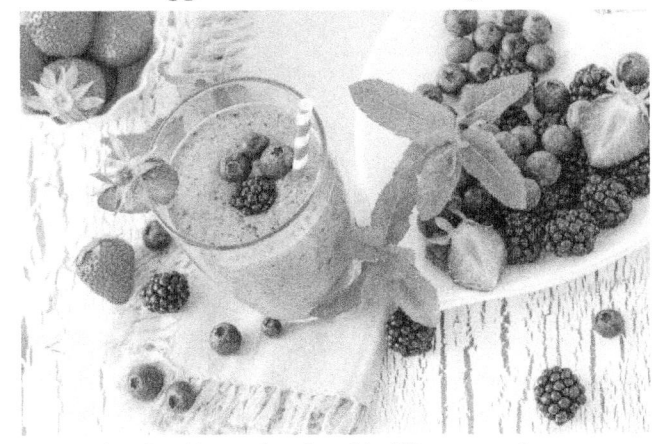

Credit: Alexandra Anschiz /Shutterstock.com

Macros

Prep and cook time: 6 minutes
Servings: 3 cups
Fat: 1.76 g
Sodium: 312 mg
Carbohydrates: 46.6 g
Fiber: 8.6 g
Protein: 4.7 g
Vitamin C: 152 mg
Potassium: 1200 mg
Iron: 1.73 mg
Calcium: 111 mg
Calories: 201

What you need

- chilled coconut water 12 ounces
- veggie and proteins collagen blend 2 scoops
- frozen mangoes 1 cup
- fresh strawberries 1 cup chopped

Steps:

1. Put all ingredients in a blender and blend for 30 seconds at high speed.
2. Serve

This is a nutritious shake which is ideal for meal replacement.

Chicken Poppers with a Fruit

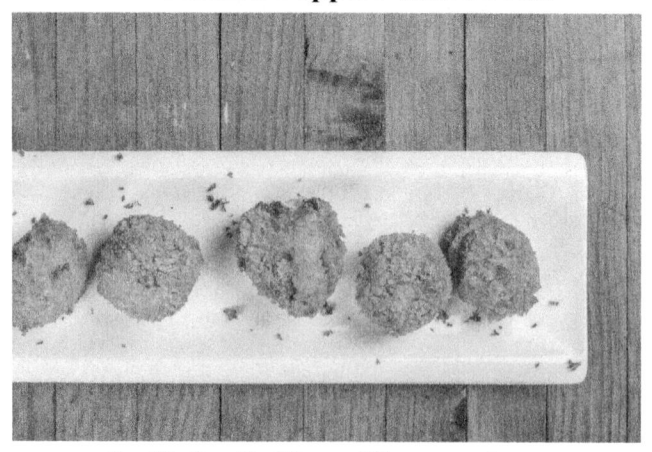

Credit: Quality Master /Shutterstock.com

Macros

Prep and cook time: 45 min
Servings: 4
Fat: 29.2 g
Sodium: 442 mg
Carbohydrates: 3.2 g
Fiber: 1.2 g
Protein: 23.2 g
Vitamin C: 4.6 mg
Potassium: 383 mg
Iron: 1.4 mg
Calcium: 30 mg
Calories: 370

What you need

- ground chicken 1 lb
- shredded sweet potato 1 cup
- finely chopped spinach 1 cup
- diced apple ½ cup
- bacon 3 slices
- 3 tsp. coconut oil
- 4 tsp. coconut flour
- ground sage 1 tsp.
- a pinch of sea salt
- rosemary 1 tsp.

Steps:

1. Prepare and heat the oven to 400°F and line the baking dish with parchment paper.
2. Squeeze the raw, shredded sweet potato and squeeze it with a cheese cloth or paper towel to remove excess water.
3. In a large mixing bowl, mix the sweet potato, bacon, chicken, apple and spinach.
4. Add seasoning, coconut oil, and coconut flour to the mixture and again, mix thoroughly.
5. Take small portions of the mixture and roll them into small poppers of about 1-inch diameter. You should get at least 20 poppers.
6. Flatten the poppers with your hand gently and place them on the baking dish.
7. Allow the poppers to bake for about 30 minutes but flip them frequently to ensure that they are evenly cooked on both sides.
8. If you prefer them crispy, place the poppers under the broiler for about 2 minutes.
9. Once evenly cooked, remove from the oven and allow the poppers to cool.
10. Serve with your preferred fruit.

Cauliflower Oatmeal

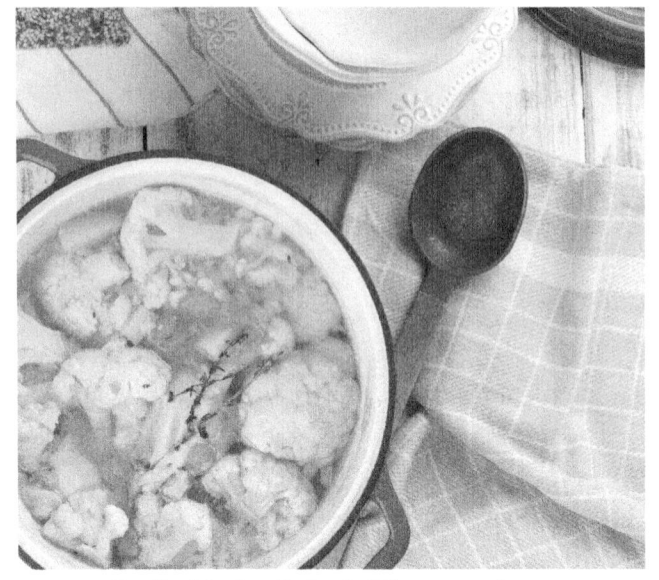

Credit: Marina Bakush /Shutterstock.com

Macros

Prep and cook time: 20 mins
Servings: 4
Fat: 8.6 g
Sodium: 74 mg
Carbohydrates: 18.3 g
Fiber: 3.5 g
Protein: 3.7 g
Vitamin C: 21.5 mg
Potassium: 324 mg
Iron: 0.69 mg
Calcium: 113 mg
Calories: 156

What you need

- 1½ cups of cauliflower rice
- ½ cup coconut flakes
- 1 cup finely diced apples
- 1 cup coconut milk
- 2 tsp. coconut oil
- cinnamon 1 tsp.
- 6 tsp. collagen powder

Steps:

1. Melt the coconut oil on low heat in a medium sized cooking pot.
2. Add all ingredients except collagen to the pot and stir until ingredients are well mixed.
3. Allow the ingredients to simmer on low to medium heat for 15 minutes. Stir frequently.
4. Add the collagen and stir.
5. Add cinnamon and dried apple toppings if you desire.
6. Serve while still warm.

Skillet Mexican Breakfast

Macros

Prep and cook time:
Servings: 4
Fat: 20.48 g
Sodium: 698 mg
Carbohydrates: 27.81 g
Fiber: 7.9 g
Protein: 33.77 g
Vitamin C: 39.7 mg
Potassium: 1068 mg
Iron: 5.58 mg
Calcium: 99 mg
Calories: 425

What you need

- 1-pound ground beef
- 2 sweet potatoes diced
- 1 red onion chopped
- 2 chopped kale stalks
- 1 tbsp. oregano
- 1 tbsp. garlic
- 1 tbsp. onion powder
- a pinch of sea salt
- 1 lime juice for garnishing
- 3 tsp. cilantro finely chopped
- 2 sliced radishes
- 1 avocado
- fresh salsa

Steps:

1. Prepare a large skillet and set the stove top to low heat.
2. Add the ground beef to the skillet and a pinch of sea salt.
3. Cook the beef on low to medium heat until it turns brown. Set it aside and reserve the fat in the skillet.
4. Add sweet potatoes and stir frequently until crisped and softened.
5. Add red onions and cook on low heat until translucent.
6. Add the kale and cook for 3 minutes.
7. Add back the cooked beef, a pinch of sea salt, oregano, garlic, lime juice and onion powder and mix thoroughly.
8. Serve while hot and top it with cilantro, radishes and avocado.
9. Preserve some in the fridge for lunch or next day breakfast.

Classic AIP Breakfast

Macros

Prep and cook time: 25 minutes
Servings: 4
Fat: 6.35 g
Sodium: 927 mg
Carbohydrates: 19.65 g
Fiber: 2.5 g
Protein: 10.34 g
Vitamin C: 52.9 mg
Potassium: 492 mg
Iron: 3.23 mg
Calcium: 51 mg
Calories: 172

What you need

- 1-pound ground meat of your choice
- 2 cups of chopped kale
- 2 cups of chopped purple cabbage
- a pinch of sea salt
- rosemary and thyme
- 2 tsp. olive oil

Steps:

1. Season the ground meat with your herbs of choice; in this case, rosemary and thyme and seasonings. Mix thoroughly with clean hands.
2. Prepare and heat a large sauté pan on medium heat, then add olive oil.
3. Add the seasoned meat and break it up gradually with a wooden spatula as it cooks.
4. Once the meat is thoroughly cooked, add chopped kale and purple cabbage, stir thoroughly and cover to allow the vegetables to cook. Note: do not let the vegetables overcook, especially if you will be storing some for a later day.
5. Season more to your liking and serve while hot.
6. Store in the refrigerator for up to 7 days.

Thyme-citrus Turkey Sausages

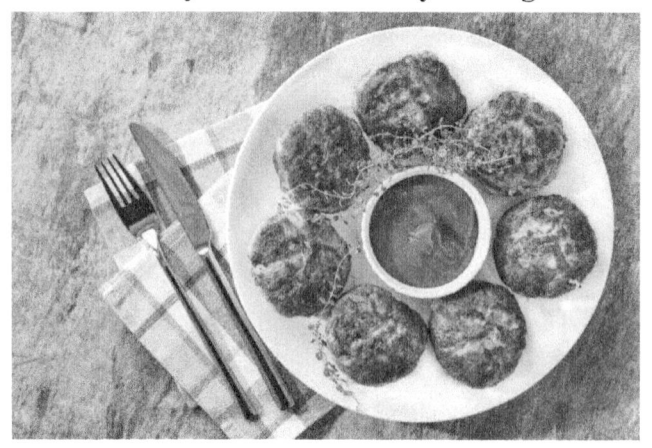

Credit: from my point of view /Shutterstock.com

Macros

Prep and cook time: 25 min
Servings: 4
Fat: 10.9 g
Sodium: 66 mg
Carbohydrates: 0.97 g
Fiber: 0.1 g
Protein: 22.87 g
Potassium: 285 mg
Iron: 1.36 mg
Calcium: 25 mg
Calories: 191

What you need

- 2 tsp. olive oil
- 1-pound ground turkey
- 1 lemon zest
- a pinch of sea salt
- 3 tsp. fresh thyme

Steps:

1. In a mixing bowl, mix the ground turkey with lemon zest, sea salt and thyme.
2. Form small round patties. You should get about 10 patties. Note: the flatter the patties are, the faster they get cooked.
3. In a sauté pan, heat olive oil on medium heat and add the patties, preferably in batches.
4. Turn the patties 4 to 5 times on either side to ensure they are thoroughly cooked.
5. Serve while hot with your preferred salad or vegetables.
6. Store in an airtight container and refrigerate for a week.

Paleo Grain Free Granola

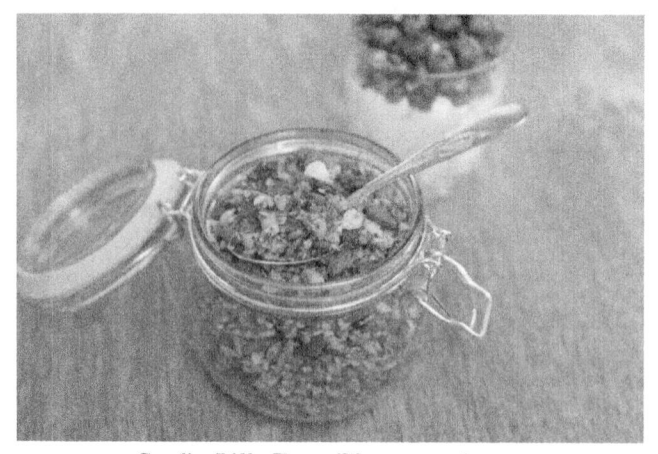

Credit: Lilly Trott /Shutterstock.com

Macros

Prep and cook time: 25 minutes
Servings: 4
Fat: 70.7 g
Sodium: 218 mg
Carbohydrates: 93.9 g
Fiber: 14.9 g
Protein: 25.7 g
Vitamin C: 5.6 mg
Potassium: 1145 mg
Iron: 6.23 mg
Calcium: 135 mg
Calories: 1048

What you need

- 2 cups pistachios
- ½ cup of goji berries
- ½ cup of sunflower seeds
- ½ cup of pumpkin seeds
- ½ cup of walnuts
- ½ cup of honey
- 2 cups of coconut flakes

Steps:

1. Prepare a baking sheet and heat the oven at 350ºF.
2. In a bowl, mix goji berries, pumpkin seeds, walnuts, pistachios and sunflower seeds.
3. Spread the mixture evenly on the baking sheet and drizzle honey on top
4. Place the baking sheet in the preheated oven, preferably on the middle rack.
5. Take baking sheet out after 3 minutes, add seeds and nuts on top of the melted honey.
6. Place the baking sheet back in the oven.
7. Add coconut flakes after 10 minutes and mix thoroughly.
8. Mix the seeds, coconut flakes and nuts again after 15 minutes.
9. After 20 minutes, the granola should be evenly cooked and brown.

Cinnamon, Vanilla Toasted Coconut Flakes

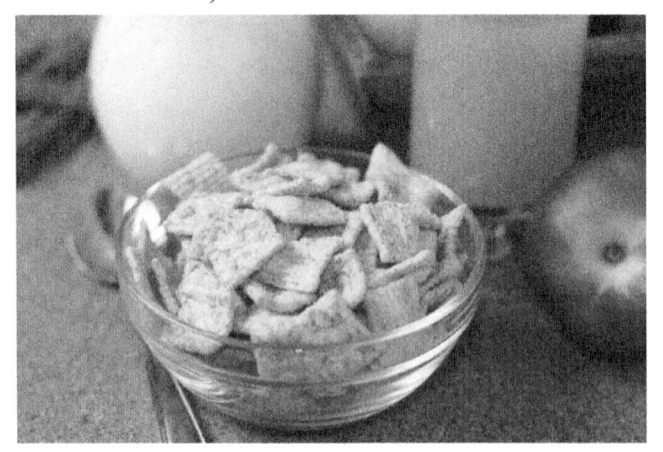

Credit: Nannycz /Shutterstock.com

Macros

Prep and cook time: 15 min
Servings: 3 cups
Fat: 32.86 g
Sodium: 242 mg
Carbohydrates: 44.5 g
Fiber: 8.6 g
Protein: 2.63 g
Potassium: 309 mg
Iron: 1.32 mg
Calcium: 14 mg
Calories: 468

What you need

- 4 tsp. coconut oil
- 3 cups unsweetened coconut flakes or shredded coconut
- ¼ tbsp. grounded cinnamon
- ½ tsp. vanilla powder

Steps:

1. Over medium heat melt the coconut oil in a large skillet.
2. Add cinnamon, coconut flakes, and vanilla powder. Mix these ingredients thoroughly to ensure that the coconut flakes absorb the seasoning.
3. Cook for about 10 minutes until the coconut flakes are golden brown. Stir frequently while cooking to avoid burning.
4. Transfer the toasted coconut flakes to a plate immediately and allow it to cool.
5. Serve and enjoy! Alternatively, store in an airtight container for later consumption. It can be stored for a maximum of 2 weeks.

Breakfast Stack

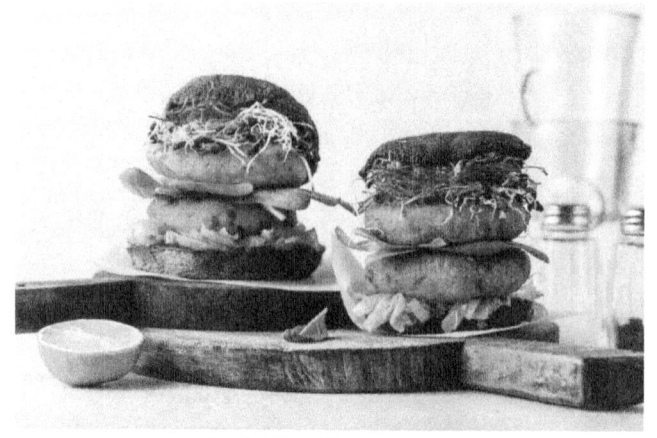

Credit: IriGri /Shutterstock.com

Macros

Prep and cook time: 20 min
Servings: 4
Fat: 75.6 g
Sodium: 235 mg
Carbohydrates: 12.4 g
Fiber: 7.6 g
Protein: 28.05 g
Vitamin C: 17.4 mg
Potassium: 1022 mg
Iron: 3.04 mg
Calcium: 65 mg
Calories: 831

What you need

- 4 pieces of AIP approved bacon
- 1 lb. ground turkey
- medium sized zucchini grated
- ¼ tsp. sage
- a few pinches of sea salt
- coconut oil (optional)
- 4 large mushrooms without stalks
- 2 avocados
- 1 lemon juice
- watercress or rocket leaves

Steps:

1. In a large, dry skillet, fry the bacon on medium heat until they become crispy.
2. Set the crispy bacon aside but reserve the fat in the skillet.
3. Blend the zucchini, a pinch of sea salt, sage, and turkey in a separate bowl.
4. Form at least 6 patties. Note: you can cook all the patties or refrigerate 3 for a later day snack and cook 3.
5. If the bacon fat in the skillet is not sufficient, add the coconut oil.
6. Cook the patties for 6 minutes per side. Ensure they are fully cooked before removing them from the pan. Set the patties aside.
7. Add mushrooms to the skillet and a splash of water. Cook until both sides turn golden brown.
8. In a separate bowl, add avocados, a pinch of sea salt, lemon juice and mash.
9. Place the mushroom on a side plate, add rocket or watercress leaves on top, add zucchini and turkey patty on top.
10. Finalize with a scoop of guacamole and a bacon slice.
11. Serve while hot.

Pumpkin Porridge

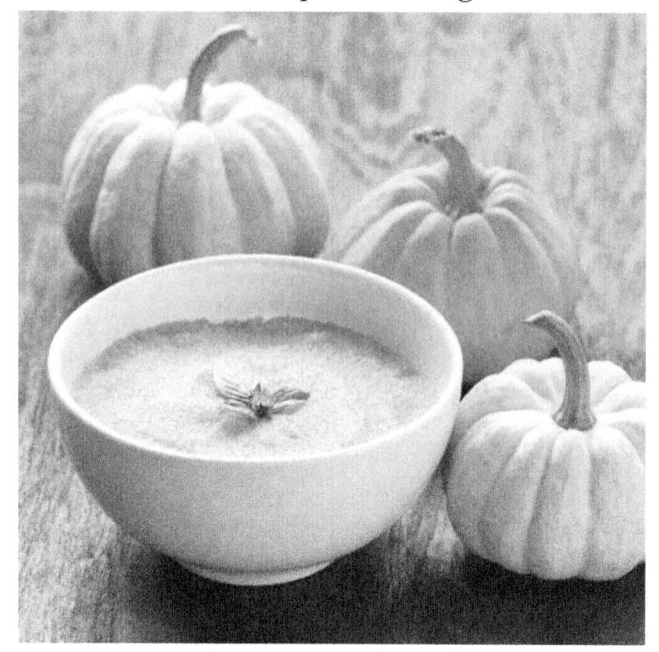

Credit: Efired /Shutterstock.com

Macros

Prep and cook time: 20 minutes
Servings: 4
Fat: 46.5 g
Sodium: 327 mg
Carbohydrates: 24.7 g
Fiber: 5.9 g
Protein: 5.79 g
Vitamin C: 5.3 mg
Potassium: 570 mg
Iron: 3.4 mg
Calcium: 35 mg
Calories: 511

What you need

- 1 can of unsweetened pumpkin puree
- ¼ cup of coconut flour
- a pinch of sea salt
- coconut milk 750 ml
- 3 tsp. gelatine
- 3 tsp. raw honey
- 1 tbsp. vanilla extract

Steps:

1. Put 1 cup of coconut milk in a small pan and sprinkle the gelatin.
2. Allow it to bloom for 5 minutes.
3. In a separate large bowl, mix the pumpkin puree, salt, remaining coconut milk, and coconut flour and stir until completely mixed. (A flat wire whisk is ideal for mixing because it leaves no lumps).
4. Heat the gelatin mixture but make sure that it does not boil.
5. Add honey and stir gently until it melts.
6. Add the pumpkin mixture, vanilla extract and whisk until smooth.
7. Allow it to rest and thicken for 10 minutes.
8. Pour into bowls and serve with fresh fruits like berries.

Cassava Pancakes

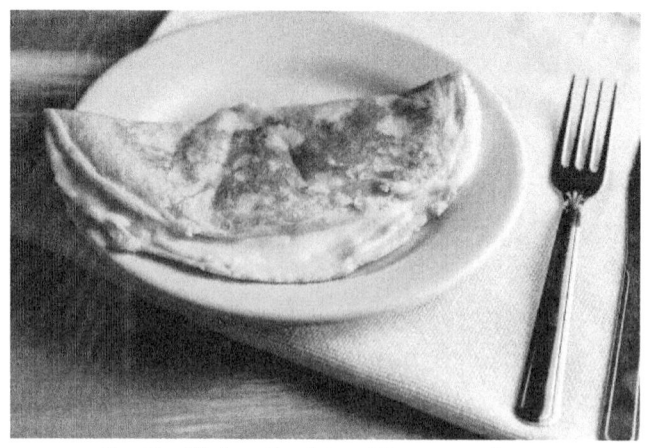

Credit: Kleber Cordeiro /Shutterstock.com

Macros

Prep and cook time: 20 min
Servings: 4
Fat: 15.34 g
Sodium: 172 mg
Carbohydrates: 39.23 g
Fiber: 3.2 g
Protein: 2.57 g
Vitamin C: 13.1 mg
Potassium: 450 mg
Iron: 1.4 mg
Calcium: 28 mg
Calories: 296

What you need

- cup of cassava flour
- tapioca starch ¼ cup
- 2 tsp. cream of tartar
- 1 tsp. baking soda
- a pinch of sea salt
- 1 1/8 cup of coconut milk
- ¼ cup of mashed bananas
- 3 tsp. apple cider vinegar
- 4 tsp. coconut sugar
- ½ tbsp. vanilla extract

Steps:

1. Mix all the ingredients except for apple cider vinegar and coconut milk in a large bowl.
2. In a small bowl, mix the coconut milk and apple cider vinegar. Add to the dry ingredients once evenly mixed. This ensures that the baking soda is activated evenly for a fluffier result.
3. Heat a large pan on medium to low heat and add a good amount of coconut oil.
4. Pour about 3 spoons of the pancake batter in the pan and flatten it with your spoon to shape it like a pancake.
5. Cook for 2 minutes then flip and cook for another 2 minutes.
6. Add toppings such as: maple syrup, blueberries, coconut cream and strawberries.
7. Serve while hot.

Tiger Nut Chocolate Granola

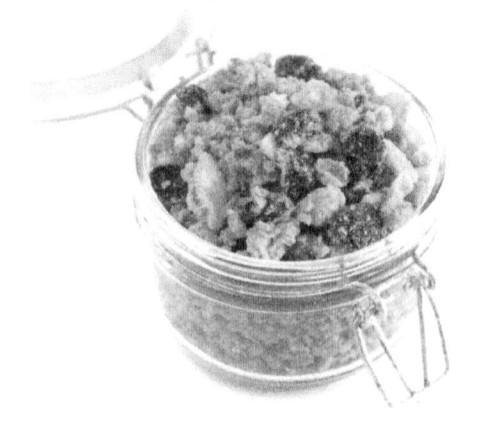

Credit: P Maxwell Photography /Shutterstock.com

Macros

Prep and cook time: 45 min
Servings: 4
Fat: 22.15 g
Sodium: 636 mg
Carbohydrates: 25.86 g
Fiber: 2.5 g
Protein: 9.72 g
Potassium: 311 mg
Iron: 0.96 mg
Calcium: 28 mg
Calories: 331

What you need

- 1 cup tiger nuts sliced
- 1 cup of coconut flakes
- ¼ cup of avocado oil
- ¼ cup of maple syrup
- 2 tsp. of cocoa powder
- ½ tbsp. vanilla bean powder

Steps:

1. Prepare the oven by moving the baking rack to the middle and preheating it to 275°F.
2. Prepare the baking sheet and line it with parchment paper.
3. In a large bowl, mix all the ingredients and spread mixture evenly on the baking sheet.
4. Place it in the oven and bake for about 40 minutes. Stir after every 15 minutes to ensure it is evenly cooked.
5. Allow it to cool and store at room temperature in an airtight container.

Coconut Pumpkin Pie Parfait

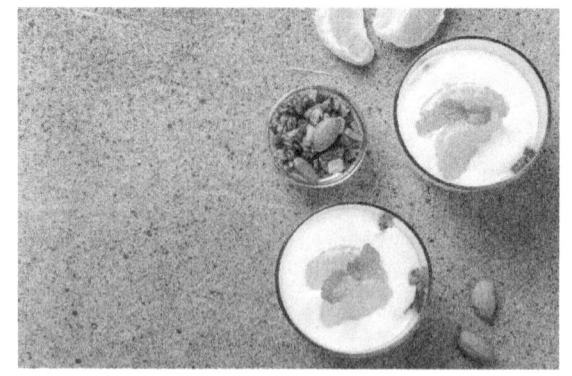

Credit: Irina Rostokina /Shutterstock.com

Macros

Prep and cook time: 4 hrs 10m
Servings: 4
Fat: 16.25 g
Sodium: 78 mg
Carbohydrates: 6.84 g
Fiber: 2.5 g
Protein: 9.04 g
Potassium: 261 mg
Iron: 2.63 mg
Calcium: 26 mg
Calories: 194

What you need

- 1 can of coconut milk or 2 cups of tiger nut milk
- 1 cup of pumpkin puree
- ½ tbsp. honey or maple syrup
- 2 tsp. gelatin
- ½ tsp. cinnamon
- a pinch of ground ginger
- ½ tsp. mace

Steps:

1. Whisk all the ingredients in a saucepan. Heat them until they feel hot to touch.
2. Pour the parfait into a cup container and refrigerate for 4 hours.
3. Add toppings of your choice and indulge!

This also doubles up as a good take away meal or snack.

Hash Casserole with Cilantro and Butternut Squash

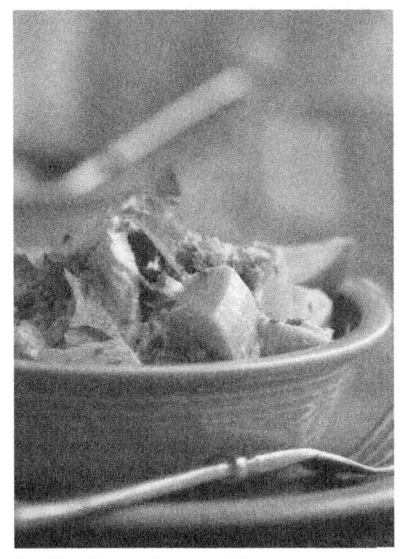

Credit: Josie Grant /Shutterstock.com

Macros

Prep and cook time: 35 min
Servings: 3
Fat: 3.14 g
Sodium: 1228 mg
Carbohydrates: 14.93 g
Fiber: 2.6 g
Protein: 1.45 g
Vitamin C: 25 mg
Potassium: 425 mg
Iron: 0.82 mg
Calcium: 58 mg
Calories: 86

What you need

- 3 tsp. extra virgin olive oil
- 1 medium sized onion chopped
- 1 medium zucchini finely diced
- 3 cups of shredded butternut squash
- 1 tbsp. of sea salt to taste
- a handful of cilantro chopped for garnishing

Steps:

1. Place a large skillet on medium heat and warm the olive oil.
2. Add onions and cook for 10 minutes or until they turn translucent.
3. Slightly reduce the heat then add butternut squash, salt, and zucchini.
4. Mix all the ingredients thoroughly, cover and allow them to simmer for 10 minutes.
5. Taste the salt and adjust if needed.
6. Add fresh cilantro.
7. Serve with a protein of your choice.

Bison Skillet with Broccoli, Pomegranate Seeds, Collard Greens, and Bacon

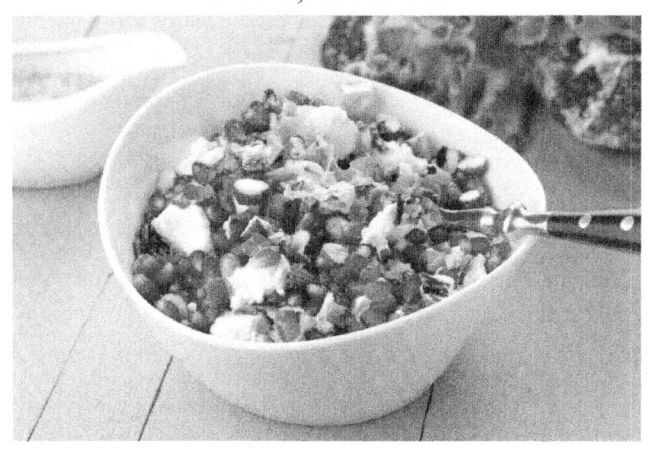

Credit: oxyzay /Shutterstock.com

Macros

Prep and cook time: 25 min
Servings: 4
Fat: 18.97 g
Sodium: 686 mg
Carbohydrates: 6.2 g
Fiber: 3.4 g
Protein: 25.88 g
Vitamin C: 24.6 mg
Potassium: 590 mg
Iron: 4.32 mg
Calcium: 167 mg
Calories: 290

What you need

- 1 lb. ground bison
- 1 cup of yellow onions chopped
- 4 cups of broccoli bite sizes
- 5 cups of collard greens sliced
- 2 tbsp. coconut oil
- 1 tsp. sea salt
- pomegranate seeds
- bacon bits for garnishing

Steps:

1. Place a large skillet over medium heat and warm 1 tsp. of coconut oil.
2. Once the oil is hot, add the grounded bison and cook for 10 minutes or until it no longer appears pink.
3. Add salt to taste and transfer it to a plate.
4. Add 1 tsp. of coconut oil in the large skillet. Once the oil is hot enough, add onions and cook until they turn golden brown.
5. Add broccoli florets and ½ cup of water.
6. Simmer for 10 minutes while stirring occasionally until the broccoli is well cooked but still firm.
7. Make sure the vegetables in the skillet are moist to avoid sticking in the pan. You may add more water if necessary.
8. Add the meat back to the skillet.
9. Add collard greens.
10. Mix all the ingredients thoroughly and simmer for 3 minutes.
11. Serve it in bowls and garnish with pomegranate seeds and bacon bits.

Banana Cookies

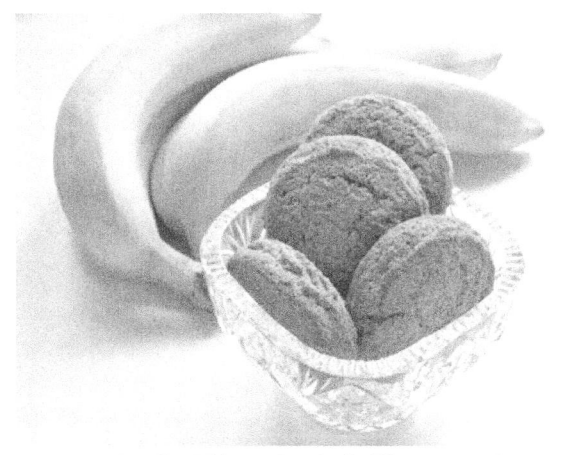

Credit: UlianovDmitrii /Shutterstock.com

Macros

Prep and cook time: 25 min
Servings: 5
Fat: 15 g
Sodium: 143 mg
Carbohydrates: 15 g
Fiber: 1 g
Protein: 0.7 g
Vitamin C: 4.9 mg
Potassium: 149 mg
Iron: 0.12 mg
Calcium: 6 mg
Calories: 188

What you need

- 2 ripe medium bananas smashed
- ½ cup cassava flour
- ½ cup coconut butter
- ½ cup coconut flour
- ¼ cup collagen
- ¼ cup melted coconut oil
- ¼ cup honey or maple syrup
- 2 tsp. gelatin
- 2 tsp. apple cider vinegar
- ½ tsp. sifted baking soda
- ¼ tsp. sea salt

Steps:

1. Rub the cooking sheet with fat and preheat the oven to 325°F.
2. In a large bowl, combine all the dry ingredients.
3. Whisk all the wet ingredients in a medium bowl.
4. Add the combined wet ingredients to the dry ingredients, but do not overmix.
5. Use a cookie scoop to mound the dough on the prepped cooking sheet.
6. Space the cookie dough on the sheet about 1 inch apart.
7. Place the cooking sheet in the oven and bake for 15 minutes until the cookies are golden brown.

Apple Rosemary Sausage Patties

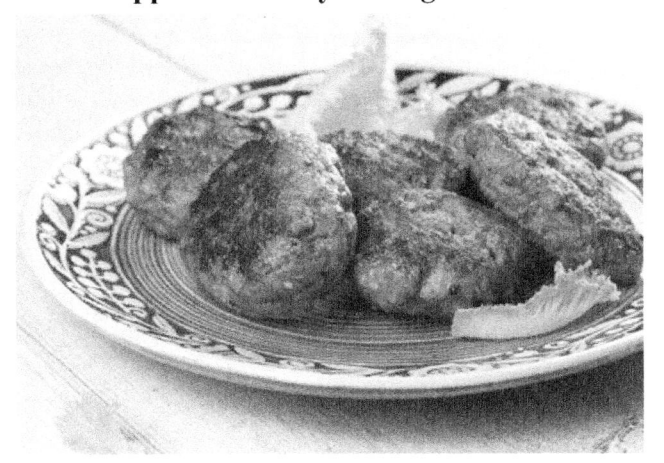

Credit: freeskyline/Shutterstock.com

Macros

Prep and cook time: 15 minutes
Servings: 4
Fat: 21 g
Sodium: 214 mg
Carbohydrates: 2.4 g
Fiber: 0.5 g
Protein: 45 g
Vitamin C: 0.7 mg
Potassium: 576 mg
Iron: 2.6 mg
Calcium: 48 mg
Calories: 376

What you need

- 2 pounds of ground turkey or chicken
- 4 tsp. of minced rosemary
- ½ cup of shredded apple
- a pinch of sea salt
- ½ tsp. of garlic powder
- 2 tsp. of coconut flour
- 2 tsp. of coconut or olive oil

Steps:

1. In a large mixing bowl, add all ingredients and mix thoroughly with your hands.
2. Form about 8 patties.
3. Add coconut or olive oil to a skillet and place on medium heat.
4. Add the patties carefully once the oil is very hot.
5. Allow them to cook for about 5 minutes each side.
6. This can be stored in the refrigerator for 5 days.

Chapter Seven: Great AIP Lunches

Butternut Pizza

Macros

Prep and cook time: 30 min
Servings: 4
Fat: 0.25 g
Sodium: 10 mg
Carbohydrates: 29.3 g
Fiber: 5 g
Protein: 2.5 g
Vitamin C: 52 mg
Potassium: 880 mg
Iron: 2 mg
Calcium: 120 mg
Calories: 113

What you need

- A large butternut squash
- Toppings like dried or fresh herbs or cheese

Steps:

1. Line a medium size baking sheet with parchment paper or grease it.
2. Preheat the oven to 400°F.
3. Peel the butternut squash and slice it into ¼ inch disks.
4. Place the slices on the prepared baking sheet and place them in the preheated oven.
5. Bake for about 15 minutes then flip the slices and bake for an extra 10 minutes.
6. Add the toppings and bake for an extra 5 minutes.
7. Note: This can also be done in a pie shell by mashing the squash instead of cooking in discs.

Turmeric Pork

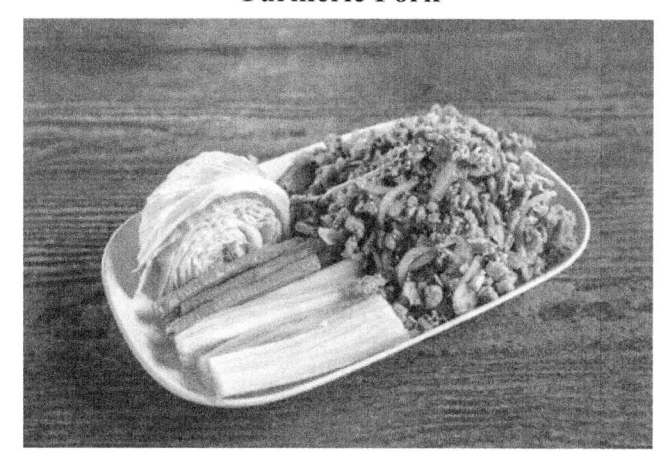

Credit: weerastudio/Shutterstock.com

Macros

Prep and cook time: 20 min
Servings: 4
Fat: 35 g
Sodium: 1230 mg
Carbohydrates: 17 g
Fiber: 4.9 g
Protein: 29.6 g
Vitamin C: 69 mg
Potassium: 940 mg
Iron: 4 mg
Calcium: 100 mg
Calories: 499

What you need

- 2 tbsp. of avocado oil
- 1 pound of ground pork
- 8 cups of sliced cabbage
- 2 tbsp. of garlic oil
- 1 tbsp. of sea salt
- 2 tsp. of turmeric
- 2 cups of grated carrots
- 1 cup of sliced scallion (green parts only)
- ½ cup of coconut milk
- 1 cup of chopped cilantro

Steps:

1. Add the oil in a large skillet and heat over medium heat.
2. Add the ground pork and cook for about 5 minutes or until well browned.
3. Add the cabbage into the skillet and let it cook for about 7 minutes, until wilted and well-combined with the meat.
4. Add garlic, oil, turmeric and sea salt, and stir until well combined.
5. Add carrots and scallions and cook for 2 minutes, or until the carrots soften.
6. Add coconut milk and simmer for 2 minutes on low heat.
7. Add cilantro and stir.
8. Turn off the heat and allow to cool before serving.

Mussels, Mango and Carrot Hash

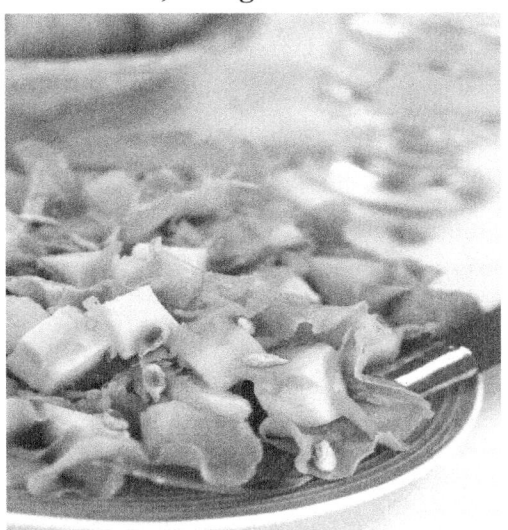

Credit: Ildi Papp/Shutterstock.com

Macros

Prep and cook time: 20 min
Servings: 2
Fat: 3.27 g
Sodium: 675 mg
Carbohydrates: 32.9 g
Fiber: 6 g
Protein: 15.9 g
Vitamin C: 51.8 mg
Potassium: 1046 mg
Iron: 5.14 mg
Calcium: 95 mg
Calories: 217

What you need

- 3 cups of shredded carrots
- ½ lbs. of shelled mussels
- 1 medium ripe mango finely chopped
- 1 tsp. of fish sauce
- 1 tbsp. of lemon juice or apple cider vinegar
- coconut oil
- salt

Steps:

1. Cook the shelled mussels.
2. Place a large pan over medium heat then add 2 tbsp. of coconut oil
3. Add the shredded carrots and let them cook for about 10 minutes until they are soft.
4. Add the chopped mango, lemon juice, mussels, salt, and fish sauce.
5. Let it cook for about 3 minutes on high heat.

Tuna Bites

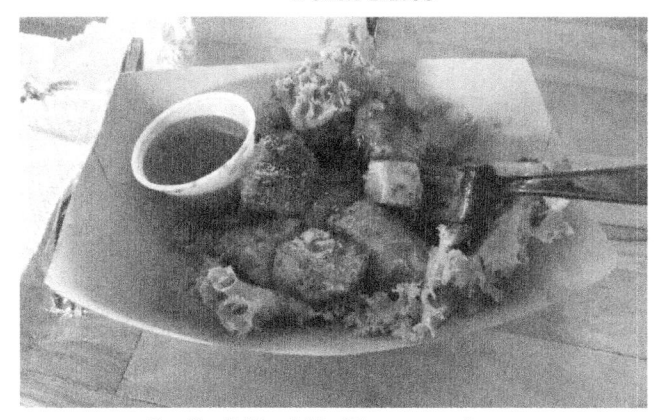

Credit: Dblock53 /Shutterstock.com

Macros

Prep and cook time: 30 min
Servings: 4
Fat: 0.95 g
Sodium: 811 mg
Carbohydrates: 15.6 g
Fiber: 2.1 g
Protein: 17.68 g
Vitamin C: 14.5 mg
Potassium: 440 mg
Iron: 1.97 mg
Calcium: 50 mg
Calories: 139

What you need

- 2 cans of tuna
- 1 cup frozen or fresh broccoli florets
- 1 medium sweet potato
- 3 tbsp. of cassava flour
- ½ tbsp. of herbs
- 1 tbsp. of garlic
- 1 tsp. of sea salt
- 4 tbsp. of hot water
- 1 tbsp. of gelatin

Steps:

1. Start with preheating the oven at 400°F.
2. Remove the skin of the cooked sweet potato and place it in a bowl.
3. Chop the broccoli into small pieces.
4. Add all ingredients to the sweet potato except hot water and gelatin and mix thoroughly.
5. Sprinkle 1 tbsp. of gelatin over 2 tbsp. hot water. Stir until it has dissolved completely.
6. Add the gelatin mixture to the sweet potato mixture and stir immediately.
7. Form 1-inch balls with your hands and place in the mini muffin pan.
8. Place in the preheated oven and bake for 20 minutes.
9. Broil for about 5 minutes to get the crispy look.

Cucumber and Smoked Salmon Ham Wraps

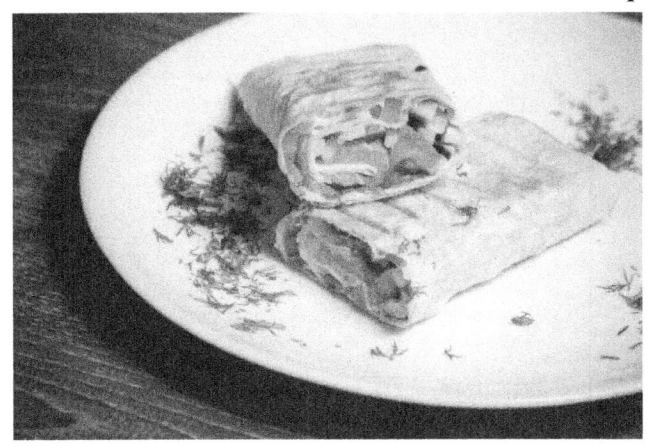

Credit: Maksym Fesenko /Shutterstock.com

Macros

Prep and cook time: 5 minutes
Servings: 2
Fat: 14.8 g
Sodium: 1890 mg
Carbohydrates: 28 g
Fiber: 9.7 g
Protein: 27.7 g
Vitamin C: 2.1 mg
Potassium: 1015 mg
Iron: 3.2 mg
Calcium: 203 mg
Calories: 356

What you need

- ham 4 slices
- ½ cucumber thinly sliced
- smoked salmon 100 g
- 1 tbsp. of coconut cream
- green salad

Steps:

1. Spread some coconut cream on the 4 ham slices.
2. Place the smoked slices of salmon on each ham slice.
3. Place thin cucumber slices on top of the salmon.
4. Roll the wrap up and serve by placing on the green salad.

Leek and Fish Sauté

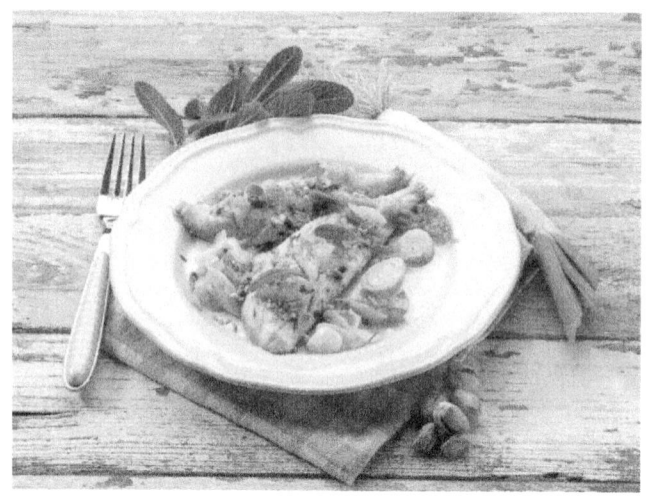

Credit: marco mayer /Shutterstock.com

Macros

Prep and cook time: 20 min
Servings: 2
Fat: 18 g
Sodium: 337 mg
Carbohydrates: 6.9 g
Fiber: 0.9 g
Protein: 22 g
Vitamin C: 5.4 mg
Potassium: 536 mg
Iron: 1.71 mg
Calcium: 53 mg
Calories: 278

What you need

- 2 diced fish fillets
- 1 chopped leek
- 1 tsp. of grated ginger
- 1 tbsp. of coconut aminos
- 1 tbsp. of avocado oil
- salt to taste

Steps:

1. In a medium sized skillet, add the avocado oil and sauté the leek.
2. Once the leek softens, add diced fish fillets, coconut aminos, salt and grated ginger.
3. Sauté until the fish is cooked and does not appear translucent.
4. Serve while hot.

Basil Chicken Sauté

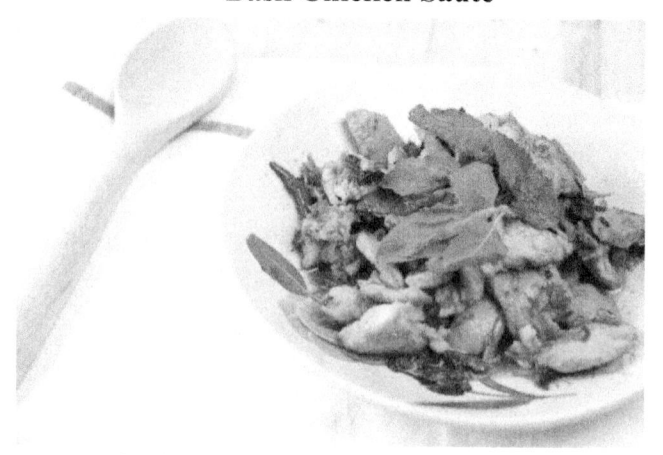

Credit: Twinsterphoto /Shutterstock.com

Macros

Prep and cook time: 25 min
Servings: 2
Fat: 13.5 g
Sodium: 157 mg
Carbohydrates: 3.73 g
Fiber: 0.6 g
Protein: 31 g
Vitamin C: 55.7 mg
Potassium: 434 mg
Iron: 1.44 mg
Calcium: 30 mg
Calories: 266

What you need

- 1 chopped chicken breast
- 2 garlic cloves finely diced or minced
- 1 large basil leaves bunch finely diced
- 2 tbsp. water
- 1 tbsp. coconut aminos
- 1 tbsp. coconut oil or avocado oil
- salt to taste

Steps:

1. Place a large saucepan over medium heat and add 1 tbsp. of coconut oil or avocado oil.
2. Add the minced garlic and cook until it starts yellowing.
3. Add minced chicken and sauté for a few minutes.
4. Add water and let it cook until the chicken is well cooked through.
5. Add salt to taste, coconut aminos and garnish with basil leaves. Mix them in well.
6. Serve with cauliflower rice and enjoy!

AIP Chicken Fingers

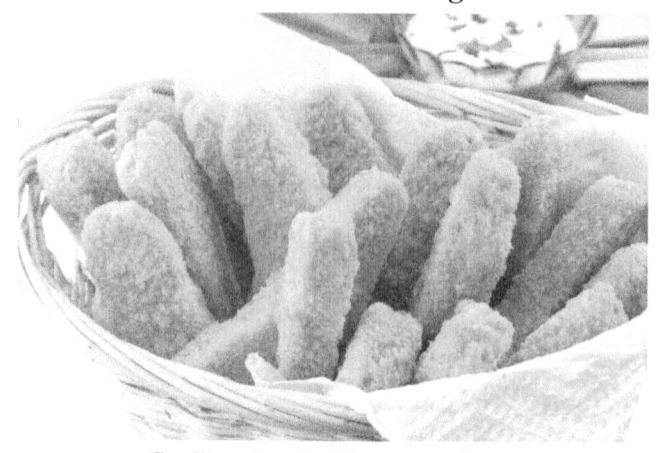

Credit: gvictoria /Shutterstock.com

Macros

Prep and cook time: 40 min
Servings: 4
Fat: 16.7 g
Sodium: 373 mg
Carbohydrates: 1.6 g
Fiber: 0.4 g
Protein: 25.8 g
Vitamin C: 0.8 mg
Potassium: 459 mg
Iron: 0.78 mg
Calcium: 21 mg
Calories: 265

What you need

- cup of coconut flour
- 2 tbsp. of AIP compliant seasoning like thyme, salt, marjoram or sage
- ½ tsp. of sea salt
- 1 pound of skinless and boneless chicken breasts
- ¼ cup avocado oil
- avocado or coconut oil for misting

Steps:

1. Preheat the oven at 400ºF.
2. Mix the coconut flour, salt and seasoning of your choice in a shallow plate.
3. Slice the chicken breasts into strips and coat them with avocado oil.
4. Put the coated chicken breasts in the coconut flour mixture and coat them well.
5. Place the flour coated chicken strips on a baking sheet and mist them with some avocado or coconut oil to make them crispy once cooked.
6. Place in the oven and bake for 12 minutes.
7. Flip the chicken strips over and mist with avocado or coconut oil then return in the oven and bake for another 12 minutes.

Green Onion and Cilantro Pork Meatballs

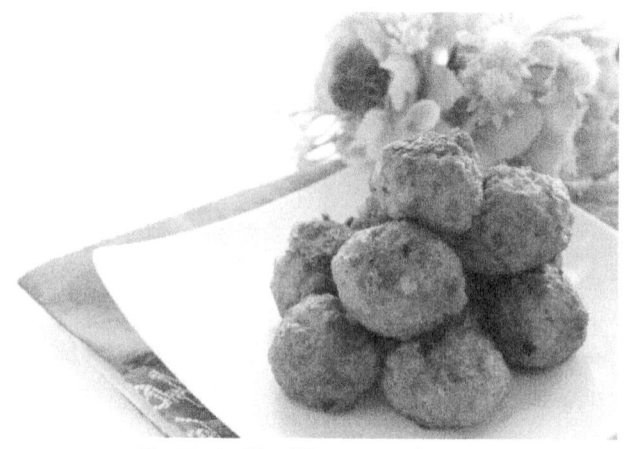

Credit: jreika /Shutterstock.com

Macros

Prep and cook time: 20 min
Servings: 4
Fat: 24 g
Sodium: 94 mg
Carbohydrates: 4.2 g
Fiber: 1.3 g
Protein: 30 g
Vitamin C: 11.3 mg
Potassium: 533 mg
Iron: 1.86 mg
Calcium: 63 mg
Calories: 357

What you need

- 1 pound of ground pork
- 1 tbsp. of garlic powder
- 4 trimmed and finely chopped green onions
- ¼ tbsp. of chopped cilantro

Steps:

1. Place a medium size skillet over medium heat and add a little oil.
2. In a bowl, mix the ground pork with all seasonings without overworking it.
3. Using your hands, shape the ground pork into 4 equal balls.
4. Place the meatballs in the skillet with hot oil and cook each side until nicely browned on all sides.
5. Cook each side for about 5 minutes while the skillet is covered with a lid so that the pork cooks through evenly.
6. Serve while hot

Bratwurst with Brussels Sprouts and Roasted Sweet Potatoes

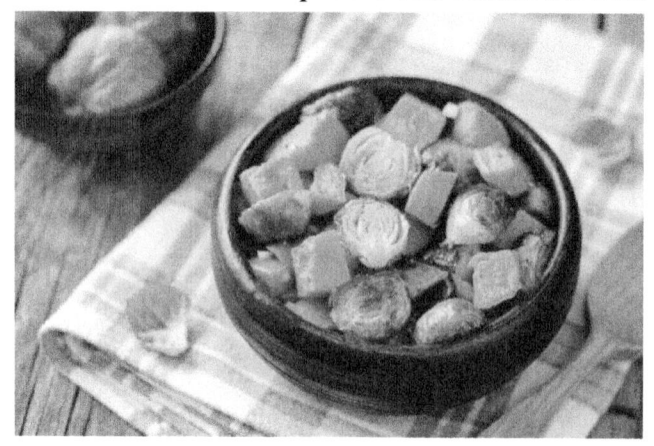

Credit: Nataliya Arzamasova /Shutterstock.com

Macros

Prep and cook time: 55 min
Servings: 4
Fat: 6.5 g
Sodium: 519 mg
Carbohydrates: 41.7 g
Fiber: 8.5 g
Protein: 7 g
Vitamin C: 14 3mg
Potassium: 875 mg
Iron: 2.9 mg
Calcium: 128 mg
Calories: 239

What you need

- 4 fresh large bratwurst links
- 4 medium sweet potatoes peeled and chopped
- 1 pound of Brussel sprouts
- 1 large onion chopped
- 2 tbsp. of olive oil
- 2 tsp. of sea salt
- 1 tsp. of onion powder
- 1 tsp. of garlic powder

Steps:

1. Preheat the oven at 400ºF and line a baking sheet with parchment paper.
2. Put the sweet potatoes in a large bowl.
3. Rinse the Brussels sprouts under cold running water and cut the sprouts in half.
4. Add the Brussels sprouts in the large bowl.
5. Add garlic powder, sea salt, onion powder, and olive oil in the large mixing bowl and stir until the sweet potatoes and Brussels sprouts are evenly coated.
6. Be sure to add more oil if necessary because the vegetables should be slightly shiny.
7. Spread the vegetables on the baking sheet as a single layer and allow them to bake for 20 minutes.
8. Remove the baking sheet from the oven and add bratwurst then return it to the oven. Let it bake for another 20 minutes or until the bratwurst attain 165º of internal temperature.
9. Serve while still warm and enjoy.

Rosemary Garlic Breadsticks

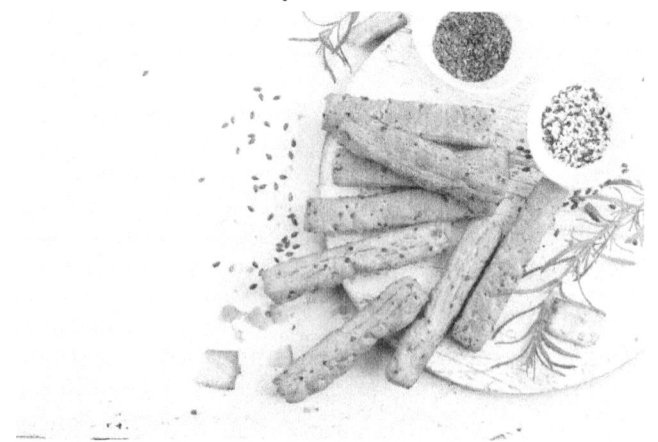

Credit: ILEISH ANNA /Shutterstock.com

Macros

Prep and cook time: 20 min
Servings: 4
Fat: 6.8 g
Sodium: 15 mg
Carbohydrates: 5.2 g
Fiber: 0.3 g
Protein: 0.29 g
Vitamin C: 0.6 mg
Potassium: 32 mg
Iron: 0.13 mg
Calcium: 7 mg
Calories: 82

What you need

- 4 tbsp. of olive oil
- 3 tbsp. of water
- ½ cup of arrowroot flour
- ½ cup of coconut flour
- ½ tsp. of baking soda
- 1 tsp. of fresh or dried rosemary
- 2 tsp. of lemon juice
- 1 tbsp. of gelatin
- 3 tbsp. of water
- ½ tsp. of sea salt
- ¼ tsp. of garlic powder

Steps:

1. Ensure the oven is preheated at 350°F.
2. Add all the ingredients except the gelatin and 3 tbsp. of water to a stand mixer.
3. Prepare the gelatin egg by mixing the 1 tbsp. of gelatin with 1 tbsp. of cool water and 2 tbsp. of boiling water. Whisk this vigorously until the gelatin dissolves completely and becomes frothy.
4. Add the gelatin egg to the stand mixer and mix all the ingredients until you get thick dough.
5. Transfer the dough to a parchment paper, divide it into 8 balls.
6. Grease your hands with some olive oil and form about 8-inch-long sticks from the 8 balls.
7. Sprinkle some olive oil over the breadsticks and season with sea salt and garlic.
8. Place in the preheated oven and allow them to bake for 12 minutes until the tops are browned.

Chicken Garlic Amino Kebabs

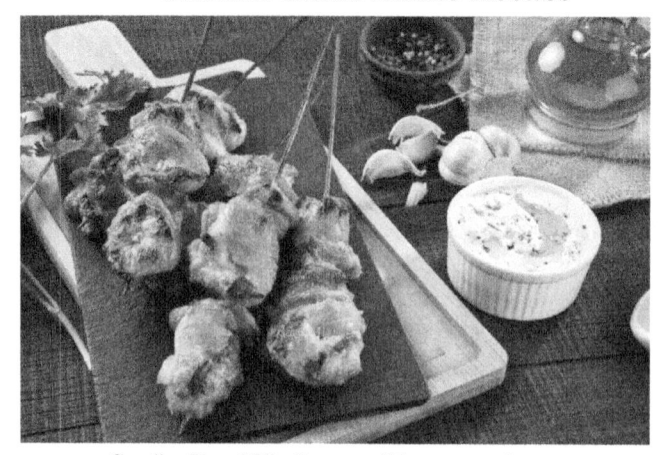

Credit: Food Via Lenses /Shutterstock.com

Macros

Prep and cook time: 55 min
Servings: 4
Fat: 16.66 g
Sodium: 641 mg
Carbohydrates: 64.9 g
Fiber: 5 g
Protein: 23.67 g
Vitamin C: 17.6 mg
Potassium: 721 mg
Iron: 3.71 mg
Calcium: 75 mg
Calories: 500

What you need

- 1 cup of pineapple juice
- ½ cup of coconut aminos
- 2 tbsp. of coconut sugar
- 2 garlic cloves minced
- 2 pounds of cubed skinless and boneless chicken thighs or breast
- 3 large zucchinis chopped into rounds
- small mushrooms 8 oz.
- 1 melted tbsp. of coconut oil
- sea salt
- 12 stainless or wooden skewers

Steps:

1. Place a small saucepan over medium heat and add coconut aminos, garlic, coconut sugar, and pineapple juice. Cook as you stir until all the coconut sugar dissolves. Remove for heat and set aside.
2. Once the marinade has cooled, add it to a container or bag with the chicken and allow the chicken to marinate for about 30 minutes in the fridge.
3. If using wooden skewers, place them in water as the chicken marinates to reduce their chances of burning while on the grill.
4. In a large bowl, add the mushrooms and zucchini and toss them with salt and coconut oil.
5. Once the chicken has marinated, skewer the chicken cubes and vegetables, dividing them evenly between the skewers.
6. Heat your grill and place the kebabs on the grills.
7. Allow each side to cook for about 3 minutes.
8. Serve while hot.

Squash Browns

Macros

Prep and cook time: 1 h 20 m
Servings: 4
Fat: 18.23 g
Sodium: 194 mg
Carbohydrates: 1.09 g
Fiber: 0.4 g
Protein: 0.4 g
Vitamin C: 5.6 mg
Potassium: 86 mg
Iron: 0.12 mg
Calcium: 5 mg
Calories: 162

What you need

- 1 spaghetti squash medium halved
- 2 tbsp. and ½ cup of coconut oil divided
- ½ tsp. of sea salt

Steps:

1. Heat the oven at 375ºF.
2. Brush the squash halves with a tbsp. of oil and sprinkle salt.
3. Place in the oven and allow them to bake for about 40 minutes until the squash are easy to pull apart and form spaghetti-like strands if scrapped with a folk.
4. Let the squash cool off. Shred it into strings and place the strings on a paper towel and squeeze them to get as much moisture out as possible.
5. Heat the ½ cup of coconut oil over medium heat and in a large skillet.
6. Take a handful of spaghetti strings and shape them into patties then add the patties in the pan and fry for about 5 minutes or until they brown on both sides.
7. Serve hot.

Sweet Potato Skins

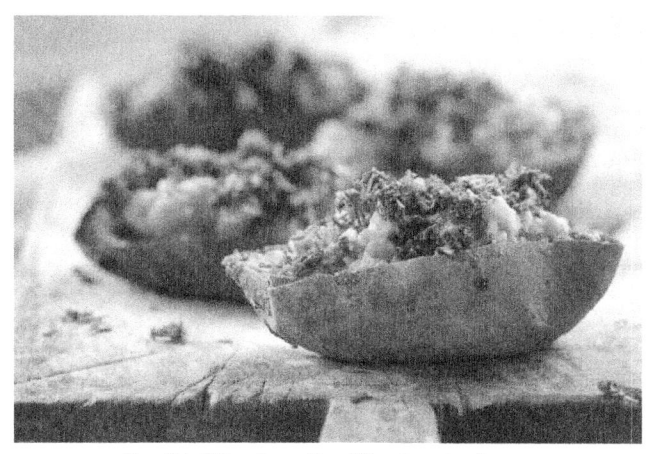

Credit: Magdanatka /Shutterstock.com

Macros

Prep and cook time: 60 min
Servings: 4
Fat: 6.93 g
Sodium: 75 mg
Carbohydrates: 7.34 g
Fiber: 1.3 g
Protein: 2.4 g
Vitamin C: 8.3 mg
Potassium: 237 mg
Iron: 0.35 mg
Calcium: 21 m
Calories: 99

What you need

- 4 small sweet potatoes
- 1 tbsp. of coconut oil melted
- 4 bacon slices
- 2 chopped green onions
- 2 tbsp. of guacamole

Steps:

1. Wash and scrub the sweet potatoes thoroughly and pat them dry.
2. Preheat the oven at 400°F and grease the baking sheet with coconut oil lightly.
3. Brush the sweet potato skins with melted coconut oil and place them on the prepared baking sheet.
4. Place in the oven and allow them to bake for 45 minutes. Remove from the oven and allow them to cool.
5. As the sweet potatoes cool, reduce the oven heat to about 350°F and place the bacon slice on the baking sheet.
6. Place in the oven and let them bake for about 20 minutes. Remove from the oven and allow them to cool.
7. Once the sweet potatoes have cooled, half them lengthwise and use a spoon to scoop out part of the innards such that you are left with ½ inch sweet potato under the skin.
8. Increase the oven heat to 400°F, place the sweet potatoes on the baking sheet with the open side facing down and bake for about 6 minutes.
9. Flip and bake the skin side for another 6 minutes.
10. Remove from the oven and let them cool off.
11. Place the bacon slices on top of the sweet potato skins, garnish with green onions and scoop a guacamole on top.

Lemon Herb Veggies and Lamb

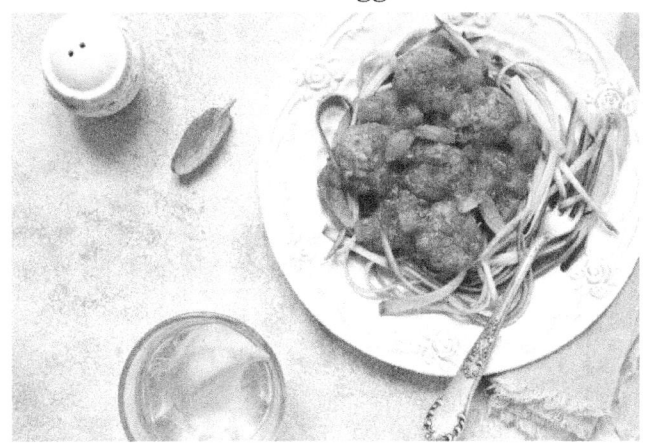

Credit: Liliya Kandrashevich /Shutterstock.com

Macros

Prep and cook time: 45 min
Servings: 4
Fat: 21.2 g
Sodium: 1250 mg
Carbohydrates: 7 g
Fiber: 1.9 g
Protein: 25.68 g
Vitamin C: 43.6 mg
Potassium: 667 mg
Iron: 1.84 mg
Calcium: 29 mg
Calories: 312

What you need

For meatballs:
- 1 pound of ground lamb
- 1 tsp. of fresh thyme minced
- 3 garlic cloves minced
- 1 lemon zest, salt

For veggies:
- 1 cauliflower head chopped to florets
- 1 bok choy head chopped
- 1 sliced mushroom 5 oz.
- 2 tbsp. of olive oil
- 2 tsp. of fresh thyme minced
- 1 lemon juice, salt

Steps:

1. Heat the oven at 400°F and prepare a large baking sheet by lining it with parchment paper.
2. Add all meatball ingredients in a medium size bowl and mix thoroughly using your hands.
3. Once well mixed, form about 12 meatballs and set aside.
4. In a separate large bowl, add all the veggie ingredients together and mix using a wooden spoon until the vegetables are coated with seasonings and oil.
5. Spread the veggies mixture over the baking sheet evenly.
6. Place the meatballs spaced out evenly over the vegetables and place them in the preheated oven.
7. Allow them to bake for 30 minutes.
8. Serve while warm.

Butternut Wedges with Avocado Lime

Macros

Prep and cook time: 55 min
Servings: 4
Fat: 15.85 g
Sodium: 442 mg
Carbohydrates: 11.55 g
Fiber: 3.6 g
Protein: 1.86 g
Vitamin C: 16.7 mg
Potassium: 398 mg
Iron: 1.19 mg
Calcium: 39 mg
Calories: 183

What you need

For butternut wedges:
- ½ tsp. each cinnamon, ginger, turmeric
- 1 tsp. of garlic powder
- 1 tsp. of sea salt
- 1 butternut squash cut into wedges
- 1 tbsp. of avocado oil
- cilantro and mint leaves
- lime wedges

For avocado lime mayo:
- ¼ cup of coconut cream
- ½ avocado
- a pinch of ginger powder
- 1 garlic clove
- 3 tsp. of olive oil
- ½ lime zest
- a pinch of sea salt

Steps:

1. Heat the oven at 400°F.
2. In a bowl, mix the butternut spices and salt together.
3. In a separate and large bowl, put the butternuts and toss with avocado oil then sprinkle the spices and toss until well mixed.
4. Divide the butternut wedge between large, lined baking trays ensuring that they do not overlap.
5. Place the baking trays in the preheated oven and bake for 45 minutes until the butternut wedges are well browned. Make sure you turn them halfway through the baking time.
6. Remove from the oven and put the wedges in a large plate and set aside.
7. As the butternut wedges cool, make the avocado lime mayo.
8. Put all avocado lime mayo ingredients apart from the lime zest in a high-speed blender and blitz until you achieve a consistency similar to that of mayonnaise.
9. Add the lime zest and stir.
10. Spoon avocado lime mayo over the butternut wedges, top with chopped herbs and squeeze some lime.
11. Serve and enjoy!

Garlic and Lime Pan Fried White Fish

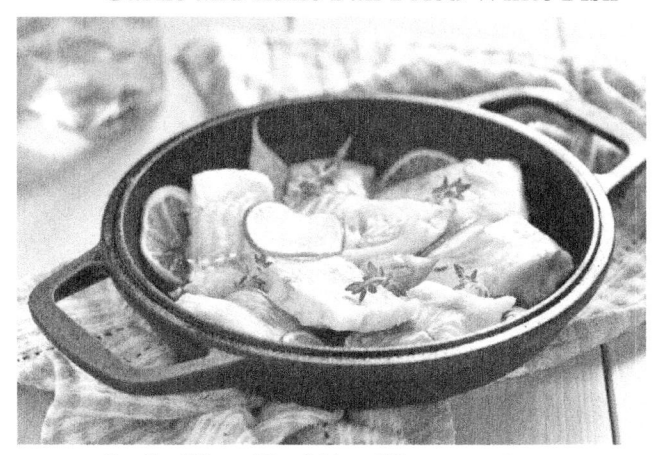

Credit: Elena Shashkina /Shutterstock.com

Macros

Prep and cook time: 10 min
Servings: 4
Fat: 20.83 g
Sodium: 74 mg
Carbohydrates: 2.7 g
Fiber: 0.1 g
Protein: 20.9 g
Vitamin C: 8.3 mg
Potassium: 463 mg
Iron: 0.73 mg
Calcium: 31 mg
Calories: 280

What you need

- 4 white and firm fish fillets
- 3 tbsp. of coconut oil
- 2 cloves of garlic minced
- 1 lime zest
- ¼ cup of lime juice

Steps:

1. Place a heavy bottom skillet over medium heat and melt the coconut oil.
2. Add the garlic and cook for 1 minute.
3. Season the fish fillets with salt on both sides and add to the skillet.
4. Allow the fish fillets to cook for 2 minutes on both sides.
5. Pour the lime juice in the skillet and over the fish fillets.
6. Cover the skillet and let the fish cook for another 3 minutes. Let the oil and juice come to a boil.
7. Remove from heat and sprinkle the lime zest over the fish fillets.
8. Serve with cauliflower rice or side salad.

Chicken Zoodle Bowl

Macros

Prep and cook time: 30 min
Servings: 4
Fat: 36.8 g
Sodium: 914 mg
Carbohydrates: 41.59 g
Fiber: 3.8 g
Protein: 16.6 g
Vitamin C: 12.2 mg
Potassium: 418 mg
Iron: 2.68 mg
Calcium: 61 mg
Calories: 560

What you need

For sauce:
- ½ cup of packed cilantro
- ½ cup of olive oil
- 2 tbsp. of lime juice
- ½ tsp. of sea salt
- 1 garlic clove

For bowl:
- 1 tbsp. of solid cooking fat
- ½ diced onion
- 3 minced garlic cloves
- 1.5 lbs. of skinless and boneless chicken thigh cut into chunks
- 1 tsp. of sea salt
- 2 spiralized zucchinis
- 2 spiralized carrots
- finely sliced radishes, cilantro leaves, avocado and lime wedges

Steps:

1. Heat the oven at 425°F.
2. Make the sauce by adding all sauce ingredients in a blender and blend on high speed until all the ingredients are thoroughly combined. Set the sauce aside.
3. Place an ovenproof skillet over medium heat and add the solid cooking fat.
4. Once the oil melts, add the onions and cook for 5 minutes, stirring occasionally.
5. Add garlic and cook until fragrant for about 30 seconds.
6. Adjust the heat to high and add the chicken and make sure they are well spread out.
7. Allow the chicken to cook for 2 minutes without stirring to ensure that the bottoms are browned.
8. Give the chicken pieces a good stir and place in the preheated oven for about 12 minutes.
9. As the chicken cooks, place the zoodles in a mixing bowl and toss with dressing. Set this aside.
10. Once the chicken is cooked through, allow it to cool for a few minutes then toss your preferred portion with dressing and vegetables.
11. Garnish with cilantro leaves, avocado slices, lime wedges and radish slices.

Chapter Eight: Great AIP Dinners

Roast Chicken with Kale and Cherries

Macros

Prep and cook time: 45 minutes
Servings: 4
Fat: 42 g
Sodium: 396 mg
Carbohydrates: 4 g
Fiber: 0.5 g
Protein: 34 g
Vitamin C: 6 mg
Potassium: 366 mg
Iron: 2 mg
Calcium: 22 mg
Calories: 533

What you need

- 4 medium chicken breasts
- Sea salt
- 2 tsp. of coconut, avocado or duck oil
- ½ glass of avocado oil
- 1 lemon juice
- ½ tsp. of cilantro
- ½ glass of cherries
- A medium bunch of kale

Steps:

1. Preheat the oven at 400°F.
2. Clean the chicken breasts and place them on a baking sheet lined with parchment paper.
3. Sprinkle sea salt on the chicken breasts and spread a tablespoon of healthy fat on the breasts.
4. Make dressing by blending cherries, lemon, avocado oil, ½ tsp. of sea salt and cilantro.
5. Pour some of the dressing over the chicken breasts.
6. Spread ½ glass cherries around the chicken breasts and bake for about 35 minutes flipping each side after 15 minutes. Ensure you check the internal temperature every 30 minutes until 160°F.
7. As the chicken bakes, massage and slice the kales to reduce bitterness.
8. When the internal temperature hits 160°F, remove the chicken breasts from the oven.
9. Slice the chicken breasts and toss kale, the remaining cherries and dressing.

Sweet and Sour AIP Chicken

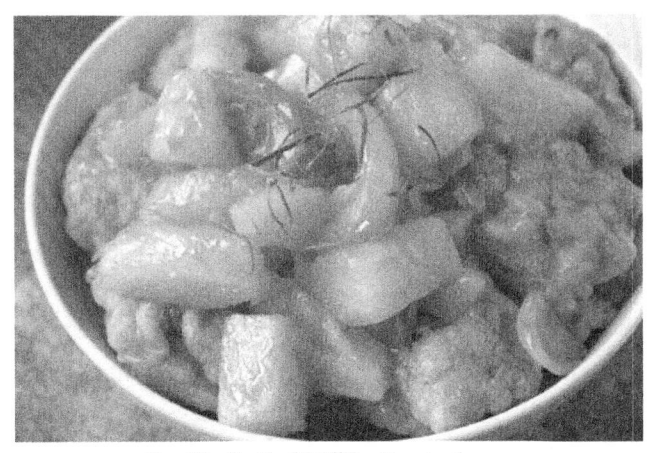

Credit: Dolly MJ/Shutterstock.com

Macros

Prep and cook time: 40 min
Servings: 4
Fat: 11 g
Sodium: 131 mg
Carbohydrates: 32 g
Fiber: 2 g
Protein: 25 g
Vitamin C: 19 mg
Potassium: 496 mg
Iron: 1.4 mg
Calcium: 47 mg
Calories: 322

What you need

- 1 pound of chicken breasts
- 1 tbsp. of solid cooking fat
- 2 glasses of cubed pineapple
- 1 small onion
- 2 garlic cloves
- ½ glass of orange or apple juice
- ½ glass of bone broth
- 3 tbsp. of coconut sugar
- 2 tbsp. of apple cider vinegar
- 2 tbsp. of coconut aminos
- 2 tsp. of arrowroot powder
- 2 tbsp. of water

Steps:

1. Place a pan over medium heat, add the cooking fat and swirl to coat the pan.
2. Add the chicken and cook for about 8 minutes. Set the cooked chicken aside in a large bowl.
3. Add pineapple in the pan and cook for about 5 minutes until they are fragrant and caramelized. Remove the pineapples and add to the bowl with chicken.
4. Reduce the heat to low and add the juice, bone north, apple cider vinegar, coconut sugar and coconut aminos. Whisk thoroughly until the sugar dissolves.
5. In a separate bowl dissolve arrowroot powder with water.
6. Slowly add the arrowroot mixture in the pan and whisk continuously.
7. Continue to whisk until the sauce thickens for about 5 minutes. Once the sauce starts to thicken, add the chicken and pineapples.
8. Serve and enjoy.

Buddha Bowl with Sausages

Macros

Prep and cook time: 20 min
Servings: 2
Fat: 27.36 g
Sodium: 1262 mg
Carbohydrates: 18.15 g
Fiber: 5.6 g
Protein: 22.1 g
Vitamin C: 12.2 mg
Potassium: 507 mg
Iron: 5.34 mg
Calcium: 112 mg
Calories: 380

What you need

- 15 ml olive oil
- 2 sausages
- 30 g of spinach
- 1 medium sized carrot peeled and shaved with a peeler
- ½ red onion thinly chopped
- ½ cup of savoy sauerkraut
- sea salt

Steps:

1. Start by cooking the sausages of your choice as per the package instructions.
2. Preheat the oven at 355°F.
3. Once the sausages are cooked, brush them with part of the olive oil and place in the oven.
4. Allow them to bake for 15 minutes or until the turn golden. Keep flipping the sausages occasionally to ensure that they are evenly cooked.
5. Slice the sausages into big chunks.
6. Sprinkle the remaining oil over the spinach
7. Toss the spinach well to coat the olive oil and serve equally in two bowls.
8. Add onions, sausages, carrots and sauerkraut to the bowls.
9. Season with salt to your liking and indulge!

This meal can be enjoyed either hot or cold.

Lamb Chops

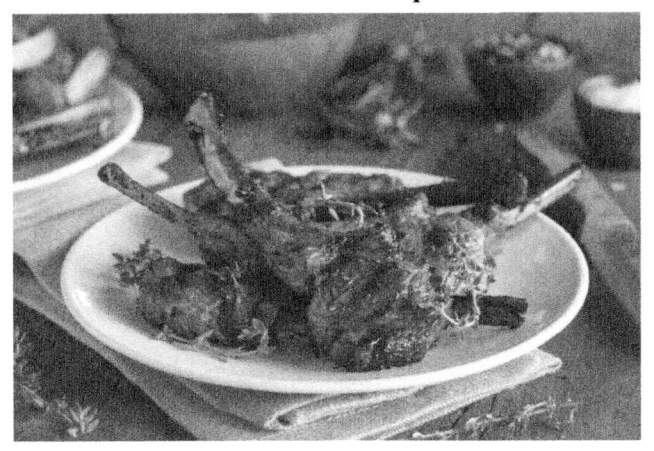

Credit: Brent Hofacker /Shutterstock.com

Macros

Prep and cook time: 30 min
Servings: 3
Fat: 16.27 g
Sodium: 167 mg
Carbohydrates: 0.93 g
Protein: 42.56 g
Potassium: 713 mg
Iron: 3.73 mg
Calcium: 39 mg
Calories: 320

What you need

- 4 tbsp. ghee that is softened at room temperature
- 3 tsp. of fresh and finely chopped rosemary
- 2 cloves of garlic peeled and finely chopped/ minced
- 6 lamb chops
- sea salt

Steps:

1. In a bowl, mash the ghee, garlic, rosemary and salt.
2. Place the mixture on a saran wrap sheet and roll it to a cylinder shape. Roll the edges to secure the mixture and place in the fridge to make it firm again.
3. Season the lamb chops with salt on both sides.
4. Grill the lamb chops in a preheated oven at 430°F for 25 minutes or barbeque them until they are crispy.
5. Once the ghee is firm, remove from the fridge, unwrap and slice into small cylindrical pieces.
6. Place a piece of the flavored ghee on each lamb chop and return in the oven or barbeque pan for 1 minute to melt the ghee over the warm lamb chops.
7. You can serve with your preferred veggies.

Pressure Cooker Broccoli and Beef

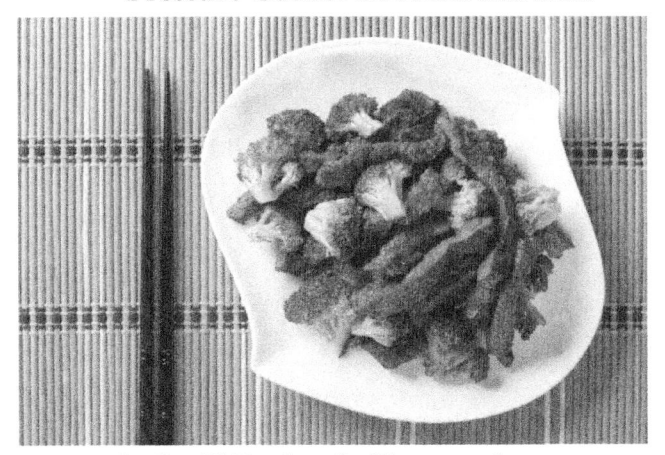

Credit: AS Food studio /Shutterstock.com

Macros

Prep and cook time: 20 min
Servings: 2
Fat: 40.9 g
Sodium: 244 mg
Carbohydrates: 4.68 g
Fiber: 3.3 g
Protein: 75.59 g
Vitamin C: 23.8 mg
Potassium: 1368 mg
Iron: 11.07 mg
Calcium: 163 mg
Calories: 697

What you need

- 2 tsp. olive oil
- 400 g beef sirloin diced
- ½ tbsp. of ginger paste
- ½ tbsp. garlic paste
- 120 ml beef broth
- 23 ml coconut aminos
- ½ broccoli head divided into small florets
- sliced green onions for garnishing
- sea salt to taste

Steps:

1. Place the pressure cooker on medium heat.
2. Add olive oil to the pressure cooker and allow it to heat.
3. Once hot, add beef and sauté until it turns golden brown.
4. Add garlic and ginger paste to the pressure cooker and sauté for 1 minute.
5. Add beef broth, broccoli florets, and coconut aminos and stir thoroughly to combine the ingredients.
6. Place the pressure cooker lid on and secure it accordingly.
7. Allow it to cook for 10 minutes and carefully remove the lid once the pressure is released.
8. Remove the broccoli and beef from using a slotted spoon and set aside.
9. Reduce the remaining liquid by half and create a sauce.
10. Season the sauce with salt.
11. Serve the beef and broccoli in 2 plates, garnish with green onions and some good amount of sauce.

Cauliflower Mash with Beef Stew

Macros

Prep and cook time: 2hours
Servings: 4
Fat: 18.97 g
Sodium: 297 mg
Carbohydrates: 14.1 g
Fiber: 2.3 g
Protein: 58.9 g
Vitamin C: 10.8 mg
Potassium: 1342 mg
Iron: 6.89 mg
Calcium: 67 mg

What you need

- 2 tsp. olive oil
- 600 g of diced beef chunks
- 1 medium onion diced
- 2 garlic cloves crushed
- 150 g mushroom buttons sliced
- 1 large carrot sliced into chunks
- 2 cups of beef broth
- 1 cup of beetroot and carrot sauce
- 1 rosemary sprig
- 3 thyme sprigs
- 1 bay leaf
- 1 medium size zucchini sliced into chunks
- sea salt

Cauliflower mash ingredients:

- 1 large cauliflower head
- 2 tsp. of ghee
- sea salt

Steps:

1. In a large pan, heat the oil and add beef in batches. Cook the beef on high heat until it turns golden brown.
2. Remove the beef once ready and set aside.
3. In the same pan, add garlic and onions and cook on low to medium heat until the soften.
4. Add carrots and mushrooms and increase the heat to high. Cook until the carrots and mushrooms caramelize.
5. Add the beef back to the pan.
6. Add the beef broth, beet and carrot sauce and herbs in the pan and allow to simmer.
7. Once it begins to simmer, reduce the heat to low and allow to cook for 2 hours stirring occasionally.
8. As the stew cooks, chop the cauliflower into medium chunks and add to a pan with boiling and salted water.
9. Cook the cauliflower until it is tender, drain excess water and add ghee.
10. Mash the cauliflower with ghee until smooth. Remember to season with some sea salt.
11. Set the cauliflower mash aside but keep it warm.
12. After the beef stew has cooked for 2 hours, remove visible herbs and check whether the sauce has attained your preferred consistency.
13. If you need it to thicken, cook without the lid for a few minutes.
14. Serve the beef stew with cauliflower mash.

Lemon Brussels Sprouts with Salisbury Steak

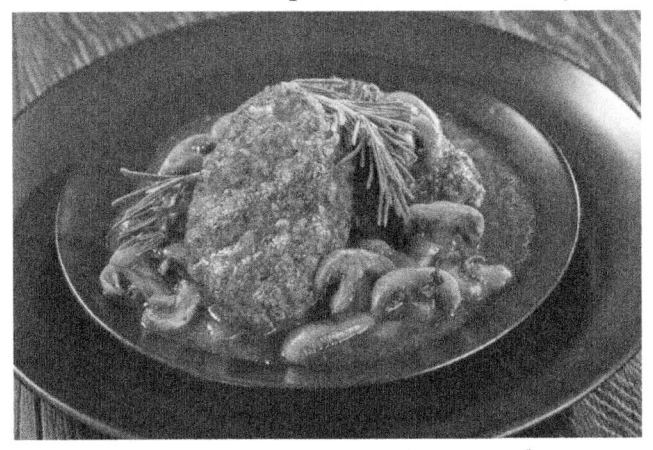

Credit: from my point of view /Shutterstock.com

Macros

Prep and cook time: 25 min
Servings: 4
Fat: 26.14 g
Sodium: 149 mg
Carbohydrates: 9.69 g
Fiber: 1.8 g
Protein: 51.6 g
Vitamin C: 20.5 mg
Potassium: 918 mg
Iron: 6.6 mg
Calcium: 53 mg
Calories: 483

What you need

- ½ kg of ground beef
- 1 tsp. of Italian seasoning or dried mixed herbs
- 1 tsp. of garlic powder
- 4 tbsp. of olive oil
- 1 medium onions finely sliced
- 12 mushrooms sliced
- 1 cup of warm bone broth
- parsley for garnishing
- sea salt to taste
- ½ kg of trimmed and halved Brussels sprouts
- 1 lemon zest grated

Steps:

Salisbury Steak:
1. Combine the ground beef, garlic powder and Italian seasoning or dried herbs in a large bowl. Add some sea salt for seasoning and mix until all ingredients are well combined.
2. With clean hands, make 4 patties from the ground beef and spice mixture.
3. Place a large non-stick pan on medium heat and add the olive oil.
4. Place the patties in the non-stick pan and cook either side for 3 minutes or until both sides turn golden brown.
5. Once ready, set the patties aside and reserve the fat and olive oil in the pan.
6. Add sliced onions in the pan and stir frequently until translucent.
7. Add the sliced mushrooms and cook until golden brown.
8. Add beef broth and reduce the heat to low-medium.
9. Add back the patties and allow it to simmer for 12 minutes or until the beef broth reduces significantly.
10. Serve the Salisbury steak and garnish with parsley.

Brussels sprouts:
1. Ensure the oven is preheated to 400ºF.
2. In a large bowl, toss the Brussels sprouts with salt and olive oil.
3. Put the Brussels sprouts on oiled baking tray and allow it to cook for 15 minutes.
4. Keep rotating the tray as the Brussels sprouts cook.
5. Once ready, sprinkle the lemon zest on the Brussels sprouts and serve with Salisbury steak.

Zoodles and Bolognese

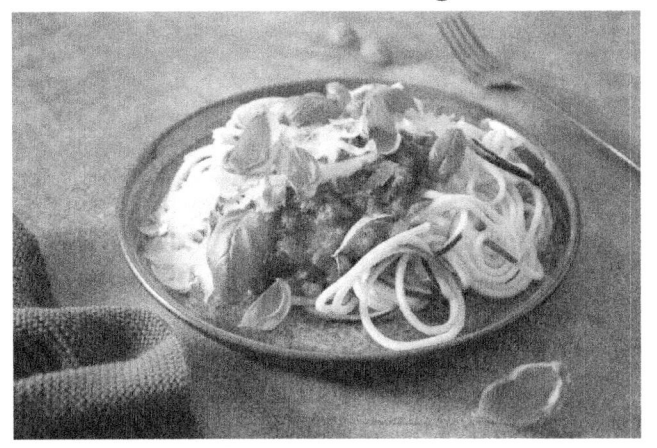

Credit: Olga Miltsova /Shutterstock.com

Macros

Prep and cook time: 1 hour 5 minutes
Servings: 2
Fat: 78.2 g
Sodium: 331 mg
Carbohydrates: 19.4 g
Fiber: 4.9 g
Protein: 56.5 g
Vitamin C: 53.9 mg
Potassium: 524 mg
Iron: 8.91 mg
Calcium: 152 mg
Calories: 795

What you need

- 4 tsp. olive oil
- 1 medium carrot grated
- 2 beetroots chopped
- 1 tsp. red wine vinegar
- 1 tsp. honey
- sea salt
- 1 medium sized onion chopped
- 2 garlic cloves minced
- 400 g ground beef
- 1 cup of bone broth
- ½ tsp. dried oregano
- 3 zucchinis shaped like noodle strands
- fresh parsley

Steps:

Sauce:
1. Heat 2 tsp. of olive oil in a medium pan.
2. Add beetroot and carrots to the pan.
3. Set the heat to medium and cook until the beetroot and carrots get soft and caramelized.
4. Add 1 cup of water and allow to simmer over low heat for about one hour or until the beetroot and carrots are totally soft.
5. Turn off the heat; add honey and vinegar and give a thorough stir.
6. Allow it to cool and puree in a blender or food processor until smooth.
7. Season with sea salt and set aside.

Bolognese:
1. In a large pan, add 2 tbsp. of olive oil then add garlic and onions.
2. Allow it to cook on medium heat until the onions soften.
3. Add ground beef and alter the heat to medium-high.
4. Cook the beef and stir frequently until no longer pink.
5. Add the carrot and beetroot sauce, dried oregano, and beef broth.
6. Change heat to medium and cook for 45 minutes.
7. Once the liquid cooks off, turn off the heat and add salt to taste.

Zucchini noodles:

1. In a large pan, put a ½ cup of water and set on high heat.
2. Add zucchini "noodles" and allow them to cook until all the water evaporates and the zucchini cooks through. This takes about 2 minutes.
3. Add salt to your liking.
4. Transfer the zucchini noodles to a plate and add the Bolognese sauce on top.
5. Garnish with fresh parsley.

AIP Ceviche

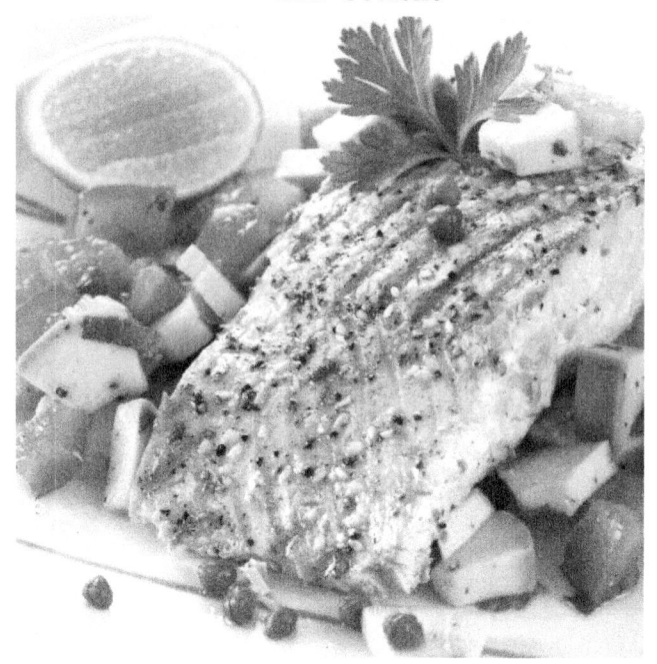

Credit: Robyn Mackenzie /Shutterstock.com

Macros

Prep and cook time: 40 min
Servings: 2
Fat: 10.22 g
Sodium: 57 mg
Carbohydrates: 10.43 g
Protein: 21.6 g
Potassium: 806 mg
Fiber: 4 g
Iron: 2.2 mg
Calcium: 108 mg
Calories: 213

What you need

- 250 g fresh white fish skinless fillet
- ½ red onion finely chopped
- juice extracted from 2 limes
- 1 small avocado diced
- 2 tbsp. of parsley or cilantro finely chopped
- sea salt

Steps:

1. Cut the fillet into ½ inch pieces.
2. In a medium bowl, add the fish, lime juice and red onions.
3. Mix thoroughly until all ingredients are well-combined.
4. Cover and refrigerate for 30 minutes maximum.
5. Add the avocado, parsley or cilantro and some sea salt for seasoning.
6. Serve immediately and enjoy!

Lime Chicken and Cilantro Salad

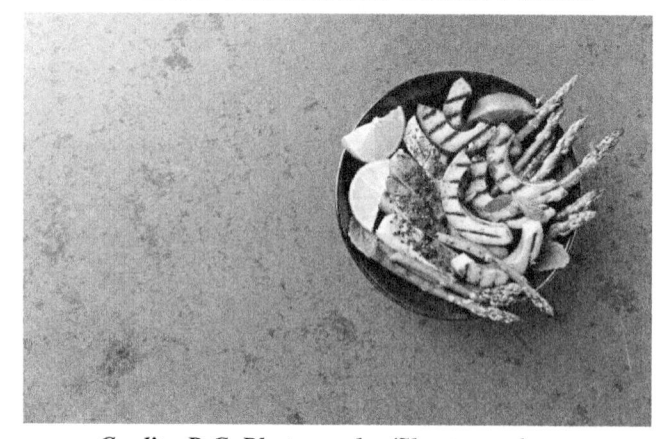

Credit: B.G. Photography /Shutterstock.com

Macros

Prep and cook time: 35 minutes
Servings: 4
Fat: 225 g
Sodium: 1500 mg
Carbohydrates: 9.41 g
Fiber: 4 g
Protein: 63.9 g
Vitamin C: 11.8 mg
Potassium: 1005 mg
Iron: 4.4 mg
Calcium: 64 mg
Calories: 850

What you need

- 1 tbsp. of turmeric
- 4 skinless and deboned chicken breasts
- 8 tbsp. of olive oil
- a handful of cilantro leaves
- juice extracted from 2 limes
- ½ tbsp. white balsamic vinegar
- 4 cups salad leaves
- 1 red onion finely chopped
- a large avocado peeled and diced
- salt
- optional: extra vegetable like asparagus

Steps:

1. Preheat oven to 180°C.
2. Drizzle turmeric on both sides of the chicken breasts and season with sea salt.
3. Using a sharp knife, make shallow incisions across the breasts diagonally.
4. In a pan, heat 2 tbsp. of olive oil and cook the chicken until golden brown on both sides.
5. Transfer the chicken to a roasting tray, place it in the preheated oven and grill for 12 minutes or until the chicken is evenly cooked through.
6. Allow the chicken to rest for 5 minutes then slice.
7. Put fresh cilantro, 6 tbsp. of olive oil, white balsamic vinegar, and lime juice in a blender or food processor and blitz. Add salt to taste.
8. Complete the salad by adding red onions, avocado and salad leaves.
9. Serve the grilled chicken breasts on top of the salad and sprinkle some dressing on top.

Roasted Herb Pork Tenderloin

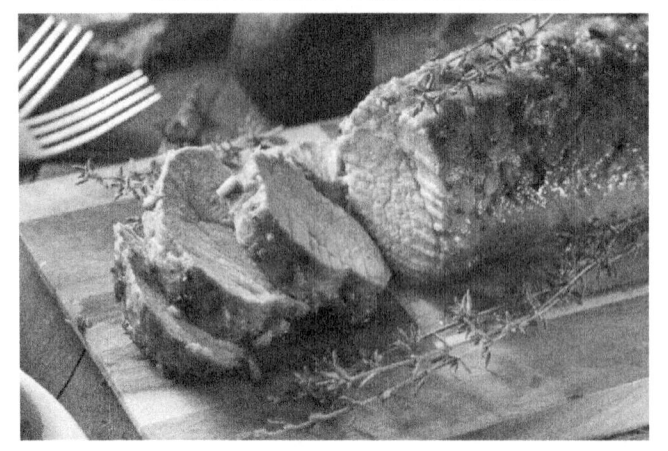

Credit: Brent Hofacker /Shutterstock.com

Macros

Prep and cook time: 30 min
Servings: 2
Fat: 59 g
Sodium: 295 mg
Carbohydrates: 4.5 g
Fiber: 1 g
Protein: 57 g
Vitamin C: 12 mg
Potassium: 875 mg
Iron: 2.55 mg
Calcium: 42 mg
Calories: 785

What you need

- 3 garlic cloves chopped
- fresh basil leaves 1 cup
- ½ cup of fresh parsley
- 2 tsp. nutritional yeast
- 6 tbsp. olive oil
- 1 lemon juice
- sea salt
- 400 g pork tenderloin
- 3 tbsp. reserved herb paste

Steps:

Herb paste:
1. Put fresh parsley, garlic, 5 tbsp. of olive oil, and nutritional yeast flakes in a blender and blend until smooth.
2. Season with salt and lemon juice and set it aside.

Pork:
1. Preheat the oven to 210°C.
2. Season the pork tenderloin on both sides with salt.
3. Place a non-stick pan over medium heat and add 1 tbsp. of olive oil.
4. Add pork tenderloin and cook until all sides are well browned.
5. Turn off the heat and allow the pan to cool off.
6. Using a small silicone spatula or palette knife, spread the herb paste on both sides.
7. Transfer the pork tenderloin to a casserole dish, cover with a lid and bake for 15 minutes.
8. Remove from the oven and allow it to cool for 5 minutes.
9. Slice the pork tenderloin and serve with herb paste.

Chow Mein AIP Vegetarian Recipe

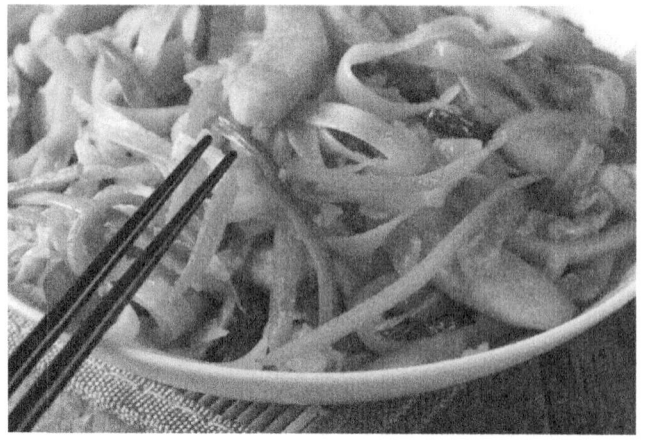

Credit: AS Food studio /Shutterstock.com

Macros

Prep and cook time: 20 min
Servings: 2
Fat: 14 g
Sodium: 180 mg
Carbohydrates: 34 g
Fiber: 2.5 g
Protein: 5.5 g
Vitamin C: 12 mg
Potassium: 229 mg
Iron: 1.8 mg
Calcium: 77 mg
Calories: 287

What you need

- shirataki noodles 170 g
- 2 tbsp. of olive oil
- 1 medium carrot sliced into matchsticks
- 99 g chopped broccoli florets
- 2 cloves of garlic crushed
- small piece of ginger minced
- 2 tbsp. of coconut aminos
- 2 tbsp. of honey

Steps:

1. Rinse shirataki noodles under cold running water and put in a pan with warm water.
2. Set aside to allow the noodles to warm as you prepare the stir-fry.
3. Heat olive oil over medium heat, add broccoli and carrots and cook until the vegetables are slightly soft.
4. Add ginger and garlic and fry for 3 minutes as you stir occasionally.
5. Add honey and coconut aminos and adjust the heat to high.
6. Cook until all ingredients are coated with the sauce.
7. Drain the shirataki noodles and add the vegetable stir fry on top.

Cauliflower Rice Pilaf with Baked Fish

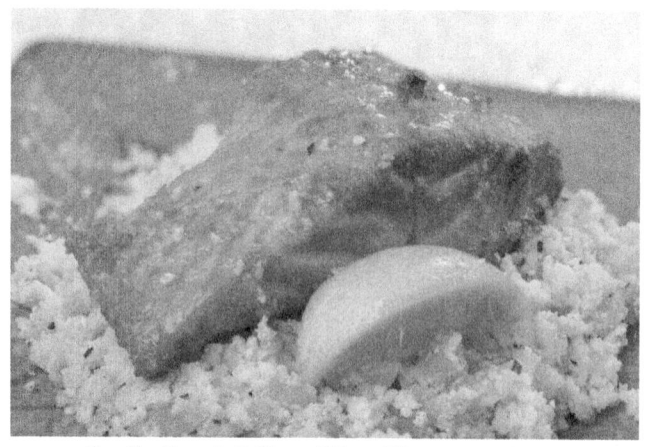

Credit: Randall Vermillion /Shutterstock.com

Macros

Prep and cook time: 45 min
Servings: 4
Fat: 2.42 g
Sodium: 121 mg
Carbohydrates: 9.95 g
Fiber: 1.9 g
Protein: 24.5 g
Vitamin C: 18.3 g
Potassium: 555 mg
Iron: 1.04 mg
Calcium: 41 mg
Calories: 156

What you need

- 2 bags frozen cauliflower rice
- 2 carrots finely diced
- 1 medium onion finely chopped
- 6 tbsp. of olive oil
- 4 tilapia fillets
- 1 sliced lemon

Steps:

1. Begin by preheating the oven to 425°F.
2. Place onions, cauliflower rice and carrots in a pan.
3. Add 3 tbsp. of olive oil and a tsp. of sea salt and toss.
4. Place in a preheated oven for 10 minutes, remove and toss. Return to oven for 15 minutes.
5. Remove from the oven and place tilapia fillets on the pan. Remove vegetable mixture off the way when placing the tilapia fillets.
6. Sprinkle 3 tbsp. of olive oil and 1 tsp. of salt over the fillet.
7. Place the pan back to the oven and allow to cook for 8 minutes or until the fillets are flaky.
8. Remove from the oven and serve while hot with the lemon slices.

Mushroom and Turkey Lettuce Wrap

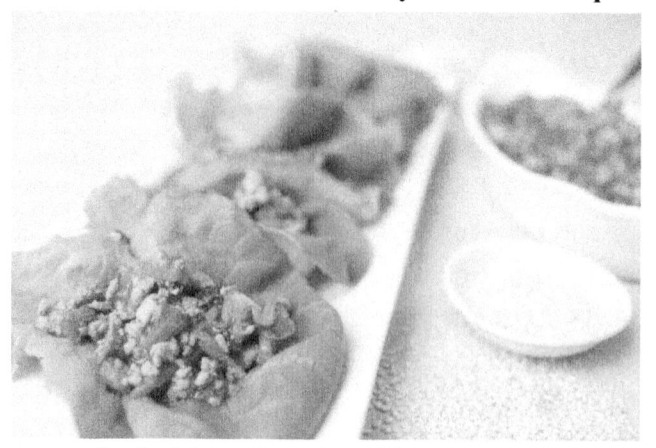

Credit: Megan Betteridge /Shutterstock.com

Macros

Prep and cook time: 45 min
Servings: 4
Fat: 9 g
Sodium: 550 mg
Carbohydrates: 8 g
Fiber: 3 g
Protein: 99 g
Vitamin C: 6 mg
Potassium: 1595 mg
Iron: 6 mg
Calcium: 45 mg
Calories: 450

What you need

- 2 lbs. of ground turkey
- olive oil
- 3 minced garlic cloves
- 4 sliced green onions
- 1 lb. of button mushroom
- coarsely chopped sliced water chestnuts can of 18 oz.
- 2 tsp. of white vinegar
- 2 tsp. of marsala wine (optional)
- 2 tsp. of fish sauce
- cilantro leaves 1 bunch
- butter lettuce 12 leaves

Steps:

1. Heat 1 tbsp. of olive oil in a large sauté pan.
2. Add the turkey and cook for 5 minutes until it browns.
3. Crumble the turkey as it cooks.
4. Once browned, remove the turkey from the pan.
5. Add 1 tbsp. of olive oil in the large pan then add garlic and onions.
6. Cook for about one minute until the onions are translucent.
7. Add wine, mushrooms, fish sauce, and rice vinegar.
8. Cook for 5 minutes as you stir regularly.
9. Add back the ground turkey and water chestnuts and allow them to cook for a few minutes until the liquid reduces significantly.
10. Add the cilantro and stir.
11. Season with salt to taste.
12. Serve by putting a few spoons of the mixture on lettuce leaves, and each as if it's a taco.

Sheet Pan Steak

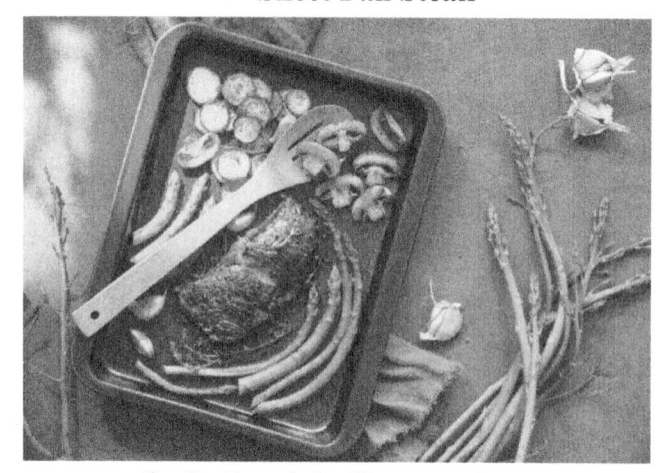

Credit: Fortyforks /Shutterstock.com

Macros

Prep and cook time: 50 min
Servings: 4
Fat: 12 g
Sodium: 145 mg
Carbohydrates: 74 g
Fiber: 9.3 g
Protein: 57 g
Vitamin C: 109 mg
Potassium: 2560 mg
Iron: 7 mg
Calcium: 100 mg
Calories: 600

What you need

- 5 medium size sweet potatoes chopped
- olive oil
- sliced white mushrooms 2 pints
- 2 lbs. flank steak
- salt
- Italian seasonings

Steps:

1. Start by preheating the oven at 450°F.
2. In a large bowl, toss the chopped sweet potatoes with ½ tablespoon of Italian seasoning, 2 teaspoons of olive oil and a pinch of salt.
3. Transfer the sweat potatoes into a sheet pan.
4. Place in the preheated oven for about 20 minutes.
5. As the sweet potatoes cook, use the same bowl as you used for the sweet potatoes to toss the white mushrooms with 1 teaspoon of olive oil and a pinch of salt.
6. In a separate bowl, season the steak with a few teaspoons of olive oil, 1 tablespoon of Italian seasonings and salt.
7. Take the sheet pan from the oven and move the sweet potatoes to one side of the baking sheet in order to create room for the steak and mushrooms.
8. Add the steak and mushrooms to the baking sheet and place it back in the oven for another 15 minutes.
9. Broil for 5 minutes until the steak top is lightly browned.
10. Take the pan from the oven and allow the steak to rest for 10 minutes.
11. In the meantime, toss the sweet potatoes and mushrooms.
12. Slice the steak and serve while hot.

AIP Hot Pot

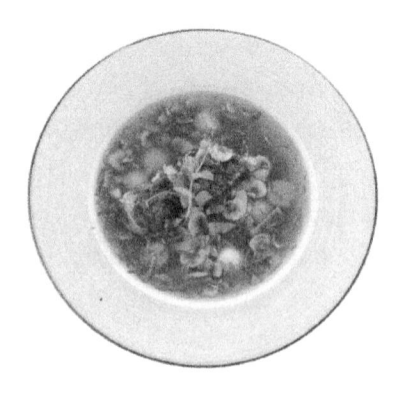

Credit: Eduard Zhukov/Shutterstock.com

Macros

Prep and cook time: 20 min
Servings: 4
Fat: 70 g
Sodium: 2070 mg
Carbohydrates: 5 g
Fiber: 1 g
Protein: 127 g
Potassium: 960 mg
Iron: 8 mg
Calcium: 75 mg
Calories: 1180

What you need

- 8 cups of chicken broth
- 1 stick of cinnamon
- fresh ginger 2 slices
- beef
- Bok choy with trimmed ends
- shitake mushrooms thinly sliced without the stems
- enoki mushrooms with trimmed ends
- daikon radish peeled and sliced
- sweet potatoes cup noodles 1 bunch
- fish sauce
- black molasses

Steps:

1. In a shallow stockpot, add ginger, cinnamon stick and chicken broth.
2. Add a tablespoon of black molasses and fish sauce at a time to taste. Black molasses and fish sauce are potent and it is easy to over season unknowingly.
3. Allow the broth to boil. While waiting, set a burner at the middle of the kitchen table.
4. Put the vegetables and meat on plates and place them on the kitchen table.
5. Once the broth starts boiling, transfer it to the burner on the kitchen table and bring it to a slow boil.
6. Remove the ginger and cinnamon stick and start adding the veggies and meat gradually.
7. Serve while hot.

Nomato Sauce Recipe

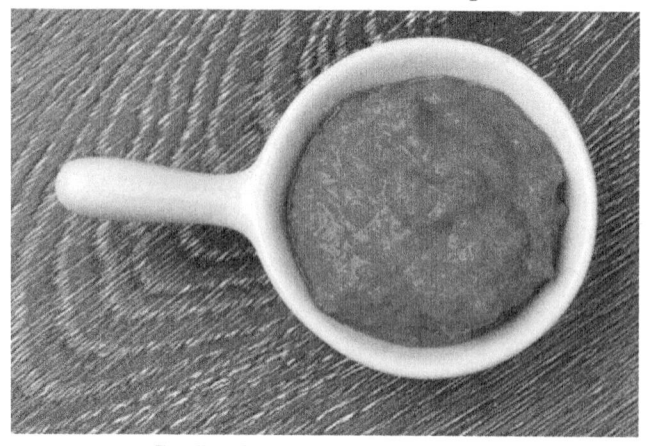

Credit: zhekoss/Shutterstock.com

Macros

Prep and cook time: 40 min
Servings: 4 cups
Fat: 11 g
Sodium: 1013 mg
Carbohydrates: 14 g
Fiber: 3.4 g
Protein: 5 g
Vitamin C: 6 mg
Potassium: 346 mg
Iron: 1.5 mg
Calcium: 52 mg
Calories: 163

What you need

- 2 tsp. of coconut oil
- 1 onion medium size
- 3 celery stalks
- 3 medium carrots
- 1 medium beetroot
- ½ cup of pumpkin puree
- 2 garlic cloves
- 3 cups of bone broth
- 2 tbsp. of sea salt
- 2 tbsp. of garlic powder

Steps:

1. Place a saucepan over medium heat and heat the coconut oil.
2. Add chopped onions.
3. As the onions sauté, chop the vegetables.
4. Add chopped beet, carrots and celery once the onions are translucent.
5. Once all the vegetables soften, add the pumpkin puree, bone broth, sea salt, garlic powder and diced garlic and allow them to cook for about 10 minutes.
6. Add optional flavor boosters of your choice like basil leaves, lemon juice or olives.
7. Transfer the mixture to a food blender or food processor and blend until you achieve your desired sauce texture.

AIP Sloppy Joe Skillet

Macros

Prep and cook time: 35 min
Servings: 4
Fat: 70 g
Sodium: 378 mg
Carbohydrates: 15 g
Fiber: 2 g
Protein: 32 g
Vitamin C: 8 mg
Potassium: 538 mg
Iron: 4 mg
Calcium: 44 mg
Calories: 815

What you need

- 2 tsp. of coconut oil
- 1 sweet potato peeled and sliced
- 1-pound ground beef
- 4 tbsp. of green onion
- 1 cup of nomato sauce (tomato free sauce - see earlier recipe)
- ½ cup of water
- 4 tsp. of coconut sugar
- 2 tsp. of coconut aminos
- 1 tbsp. of apple cider vinegar
- ½ tbsp. of garlic powder
- a pinch of sea salt

Steps:

1. Place a large skillet over medium heat and melt the coconut oil.
2. Add the sweet potatoes and sauté for 10 minutes until they soften.
3. Set the sweet potatoes aside and drain the fat from the skillet.
4. Add onions and ground beef to the skillet and sauté on medium heat.
5. Break the ground beef with a wooden spatula and stir until completely browned.
6. Remove the beef from the heat and drain excess fat from the skillet.
7. To make the sauce, put the nomato sauce, water, coconut sugar, coconut aminos, apple cider vinegar, garlic powder, and a pinch of salt to the blender and blend on high speed until smooth.
8. Add back the sweet potatoes and combine with the sauce. Stir until thoroughly combined and allow it to simmer for 10 minutes.
9. Turn off the heat and add green onions.
10. Season further to your liking and allow it to cool before serving.

Ginger Cream Sauce with Ground Pork

Macros

Prep and cook time: 30 min
Servings: 4
Fat: 82 g
Sodium: 238 mg
Carbohydrates: 23 g
Fiber: 7 g
Protein: 47 g
Vitamin C: 5 mg
Potassium: 1094 mg
Iron: 5 mg
Calcium: 141 mg
Calories: 982

What you need

- 1 pound of ground pork
- 2 tbsp. of coconut oil
- 1 medium white onion diced
- 2 garlic cloves minced
- 3 tsp. of ginger grated
- coleslaw mix 12 oz.
- 2 tbsp. of apple cider vinegar
- 8 tsp. of coconut aminos
- 4 tsp. of chopped green onions
- ¼ cup of coconut cream
- sea salt

Steps:

1. Place a large skillet over medium heat, add the pork and season lightly with salt.
2. Once the pork has browned set it aside and drain the fat from the skillet.
3. Add coconut oil to the skillet and sauté the ginger, onions and garlic until translucent.
4. All the apple cider vinegar, coleslaw mix, and coconut aminos.
5. Season with salt and stir to combine all ingredients. Sauté for 5 minutes.
6. Add back the pork and stir thoroughly. Allow to cook for about a minute.
7. Turn off the heat and garnish with green onions.
8. Serve with sauce.
9. To make the sauce; add the coconut cream, coconut aminos, 1 tsp. of apple cider vinegar, 2 tsp. of grated ginger and a pinch of salt in a bowl and combine thoroughly.

AIP Unstuffed Cabbage Roll

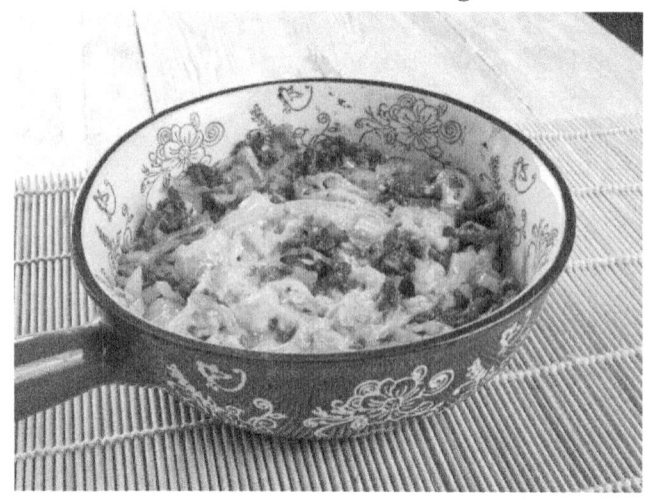

Credit: Fanfo /Shutterstock.com

Macros

Prep and cook time: 35 min
Servings: 4
Fat: 13.6 g
Sodium: 2500 mg
Carbohydrates: 32 g
Fiber: 9.3 g
Protein: 35 g
Vitamin C: 41 mg
Potassium: 990 mg
Iron: 4.6 mg
Calcium: 62 mg
Calories: 408

What you need

- 1 pound of ground beef
- 1 onion diced
- 2 minced garlic cloves
- 1 cup of cauliflower pre-riced or riced using with food processor
- 1 green cabbage chopped
- ½ cup of beef broth
- 2 cups of nomato sauce
- a pinch of sea salt
- 1 tbsp. of parsley

Steps:

1. In a large pan, cook the ground beef on medium heat until browned.
2. Once browned, remove the beef from the pan and set aside. Reserve the fat.
3. Add onions and garlic in the pan and sauté for 5 minutes.
4. Add riced cauliflower to the pan and allow it to cook for 8 minutes until soft.
5. Add back the cooked ground beef, nomato sauce, salt, cabbage slices, and beef broth.
6. Stir to combine and allow it to simmer for 15 minutes.
7. Turn off the heat and serve the unstuffed cabbage roll while still warm.

AIP Spaghetti Squash Pizza Casserole

Macros

Prep and cook time: 50 min
Servings: 4
Fat: 15 g
Sodium: 620 mg
Carbohydrates: 15 g
Fiber: 2.7 g
Protein: 29.4 g
Vitamin C: 15.4 mg
Potassium: 821 mg
Iron: 5 mg
Calcium: 80 mg
Calories: 310

What you need

- 1 spaghetti squash cooked
- 1 pound of ground beef
- 1 small white onion diced
- 2 minced garlic cloves
- 1 cup of sliced mushrooms
- sea salt 1 tsp.
- 1 cup of sugar free nomato sauce that is AIP friendly

Toppings:
- ¼ cup of sliced black olives
- ¼ cup of diced red onions
- 2 tsp. of chopped basil
- 1 tbsp. of chopped parsley

Steps:

1. Prepare a baking dish of about 8" x 8" size and preheat the oven at 400°F.
2. Place a large skillet over medium heat and add the ground beef and a pinch of salt.
3. Allow the beef to brown evenly and set it aside. Reserve the fat in the skillet.
4. Add garlic and white onions to the pan and sauté for a few minutes until the onions are translucent.
5. Add mushrooms and cook for 5 minutes until they soften. Set it aside.
6. Put the cooked spaghetti squash strands in a large mixing bowl and pat down excess liquid with a clean cloth or paper towel.
7. Mix the cooked vegetables, ground beef and 1 cup of sauce with the spaghetti squash. Pour this in a casserole dish. (Retain 8 mushroom pieces).
8. Top the casserole with the remaining mushrooms and sauce.
9. Place in preheated oven and allow it to bake for 30 minutes.
10. Remove from the oven, add toppings and serve!

Chapter Nine: Easy AIP Salad and Soup Recipes

AIP Salad Recipes

Mediterranean Tuna Salad

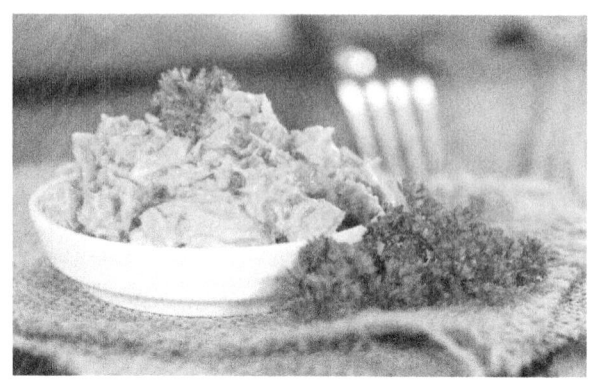

Credit: HandmadePictures /Shutterstock.com

Macros

Prep and cook time: 10 min
Servings: 2
Fat: 26 g
Sodium: 4300 mg
Carbohydrates: 7.2 g
Fiber: 4.3 g
Protein: 308 g
Vitamin C: 13.2 mg
Potassium: 3000 mg
Iron: 26.5 mg
Calcium: 297 mg
Calories: 1450

What you need

- ½ cup artichokes cooked, diced and drained
- 10 pitted and diced olives
- 2 cans of flaked tuna
- 2 celery ribs finely diced
- 3 tbsp. olive oil
- 2 garlic cloves minced
- 3 tbsp. parsley finely chopped
- 1 tsp. lemon juice
- a pinch of sea salt

Steps:

1. In a large bowl, combine all ingredients and mix thoroughly.
2. Serve and enjoy!

Shredded Chicken Salad (Vietnamese)

Macros

Prep and cook time: 40 min
Servings: 4
Fat: 7.5 g
Sodium: 153 mg
Carbohydrates: 8.5 g
Fiber: 2.5 g
Protein: 1.9 g
Vitamin C: 10.5 mg
Potassium: 433 mg
Iron: 0.8 mg
Calcium: 52 mg
Calories: 105

What you need

- 1 small red onion thinly diced
- 2 medium carrots grated or cut into matchsticks
- small piece of cucumber about ¼ inch long
- 3.5-inch-thick daikon piece grated or julienned
- 4 large chicken thighs
- 1 cup of chopped cilantro
- ½ cup of chopped mint leaves
- ½ tbsp. fish sauce
- 2 minced garlic cloves
- 2 tsp. apple cider vinegar
- ½ grated ginger
- 2 tsp. avocado oil
- 2 tsp. coconut aminos

Steps:

1. Set the oven at 375ºF.
2. Place a large ovenproof pan on medium heat and heat until very hot.
3. Put the chicken thighs in the hot pan.
4. Let it cook undisturbed for 6 minutes or until the chicken gets a deep golden brown color. Trying to move the chicken thighs before they are cooked rips off the skin stuck in the pan.
5. Once the skin is browned, transfer the chicken pieces to a plate. Discard the rendered fat or store it for later use.
6. Add back the chicken pieces to the pan with the skin side facing up.
7. Place the pan in the preheated oven and allow the chicken to cook for 15 minutes.
8. Remove the chicken and transfer to a clean plate. Allow it to cool before serving.
9. As it cools, prepare the dressing by putting 2 minced garlic cloves, ½ tbsp. fish sauce, 2 minced garlic cloves, ½ grated ginger, 2 tsp. avocado oil, and 2 tsp. coconut aminos in a bowl and mix thoroughly.
10. Cut the chicken into small pieces.
11. Place the salad ingredients in a bowl and drizzle the dressing. Mix thoroughly.
12. Serve the salad in four plates and place the chicken pieces on top.
13. Serve while still warm.

Brussels Sprout

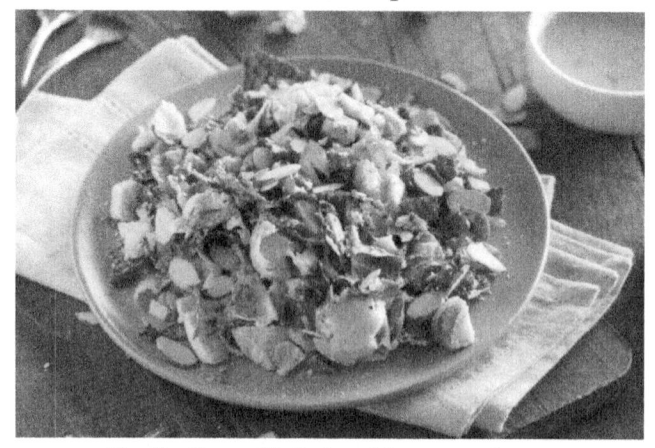

Credit: Brent Hofacker /Shutterstock.com

Macros

Prep and cook time: 20 min
Servings: 4
Fat: 10.7 g
Sodium: 368 mg
Carbohydrates: 21.3 g
Fiber: 7.6 g
Protein: 5.3 g
Vitamin C: 133 mg
Potassium: 930 mg
Iron: 2.5 mg
Calcium: 103 mg
Calories: 187

What you need

- 1 lb. of Brussels sprouts without ends and thinly sliced
- 6 tsp. of olive oil
- ½ tsp. of sea salt
- 1 small red onion sliced
- radishes 1 bunch
- 1 fennel bulb
- 1 mandarin orange
- 1 small lemon for juicing
- 2 tsp. of champagne vinegar
- 1 tsp. of ginger powder

Steps:

1. In a large bowl, put sprouts in first, then salt and oil.
2. Mix thoroughly for about 5 minutes with your hands. Ensure tough fibers are broken down.
3. Add the radishes, onions, oranges, and fennel to the bowl and mix all ingredients well.
4. Add the ginger powder, vinegar and lemon juice in a separate small bowl.
5. Whisk until well combined and add to the salad.
6. Toss to combine and serve.

Avocado Salad

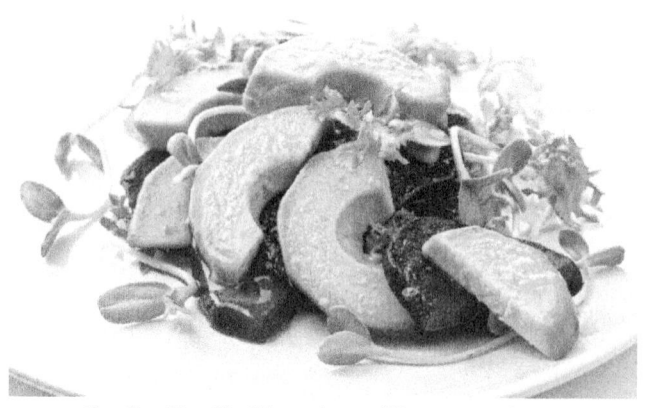

Credit: Natalia Lisovskaya /Shutterstock.com

Macros

Prep and cook time: 10 min
Servings: 2
Fat: 15 g
Sodium: 42 mg
Carbohydrates: 14 g
Fiber: 7 g
Protein: 2.5 g
Vitamin C: 21.8 mg
Potassium: 575 mg
Iron: 0.73 mg
Calcium: 25 mg
Calories: 182

What you need

- ½ red onion sliced thinly
- 2 tsp. of red wine vinegar
- 1 big avocado sliced
- 1 small cooked and pickled beetroot
- 1 small carrot sliced like matchsticks
- freshly squeezed lemon juice
- olive oil
- chives

Steps:

1. Add red wine vinegar and red onions in a bowl and set aside to pickle as you prepare the other ingredients.
2. Add lemon juice and salt to the diced avocado and give one good stir.
3. Put some avocado, carrots and beets on two plates and sprinkle some olive oil.
4. Add the now pickled onions on top of the salad and the remaining vinegar as well.
5. Add chives for garnishing and serve immediately.

Winter Salad

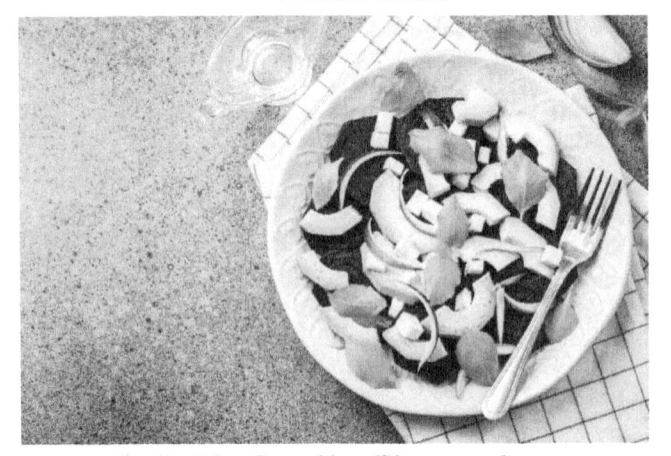

Credit: Irina Rostokina /Shutterstock.com

Macros

Prep and cook time: 60 min
Servings: 4
Fat: 22 g
Sodium: 25 mg
Carbohydrates: 16 g
Fiber: 5 g
Protein: 2.3 g
Vitamin C: 15 mg
Potassium: 506 mg
Iron: 1 mg
Calcium: 43 mg
Calories: 254

What you need

- 1 big beetroot
- 2 medium sweet potatoes
- arugula 2 cups
- 1 sliced avocado
- olive oil 60 ml
- 4 tsp. of balsamic vinegar
- 1 tsp. of maple syrup or honey

Steps:

1. Preheat the oven at 200ºC.
2. Clean the sweet potatoes and beetroot then wrap them in foil.
3. Bake the sweet potatoes and beetroot for one hour or until they are tender.
4. Rinse under cold water and peel.
5. Slice the cooked sweet potatoes and beetroot into cubes.
6. Whisk the 60 ml olive oil, 1 tsp. of maple syrup or honey and 4 tsp. of balsamic vinegar together to make the dressing.
7. Toss the dressing with the salad ingredients and serve.

Waldorf Salad

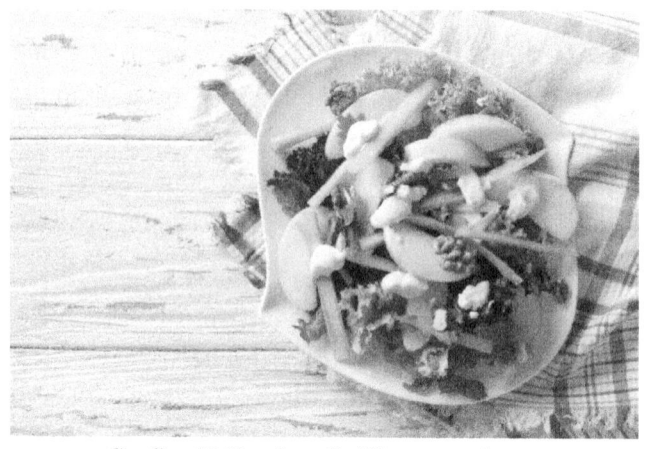

Credit: AS Food studio/Shutterstock.com

Macros

Prep and cook time: 10 min
Servings: 2
Fat: 12.7 g
Sodium: 68 mg
Carbohydrates: 55 g
Fiber: 19.2 g
Protein: 10 g
Vitamin C: 29.9 mg
Potassium: 1987 mg
Iron: 7.22 mg
Calcium: 230 mg
Calories: 340

What you need

- 2 tbsp. of refrigerated coconut cream
- 1 tsp. of lemon juice
- 1 green or granny smith apple thinly sliced
- 1 celery stalk sliced thinly
- 10 halved grapes
- 1 romaine lettuce head chopped
- salt

Steps:

1. Start by making the salad dressing; mix lemon juice, coconut cream and a pinch of salt.
2. In a large bowl, add all the other ingredients and mix.
3. Add the salad dressing and toss to ensure all ingredients are well coated.

Bacon, Salmon and Pesto Salad

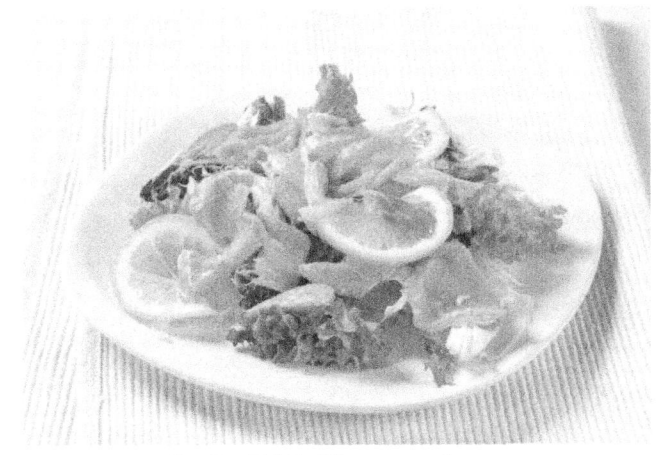

Credit: Tobik /Shutterstock.com

Macros

Prep and cook time: 15 min
Servings: 4
Fat: 9.3 g
Sodium: 75 mg
Carbohydrates: 1.89 g
Fiber: 0.5 g
Protein: 29.4 g
Vitamin C: 8.3 mg
Potassium: 795 mg
Iron: 1.46 mg
Calcium: 31 mg
Calories: 215

What you need

- 1 packet of smoked wild salmon
- 4 nitrate free and sugar free bacon slices
- 4 cups of greens or lettuce
- dairy free pesto 2 tbsp.
- a pinch each of thyme and chives
- freshly squeezed lemon juice

Steps:

1. Prepare a baking sheet and line it with parchment paper.
2. Preheat the oven at 350°F.
3. Add the bacon slices to the baking sheet and allow to bake for 15 minutes or until crispy. Set them aside once ready.
4. Prepare the salad in a large bowl. Mix the greens or lettuce with chives and thyme, add pesto and mix thoroughly until the greens or lettuce are well coated.
5. Place the wild smoked salmon on top and drizzle the remaining herbs and pesto. Add lemon juice and the crispy bacon bites.
6. Serve and indulge!

Lemon Tuna Salad

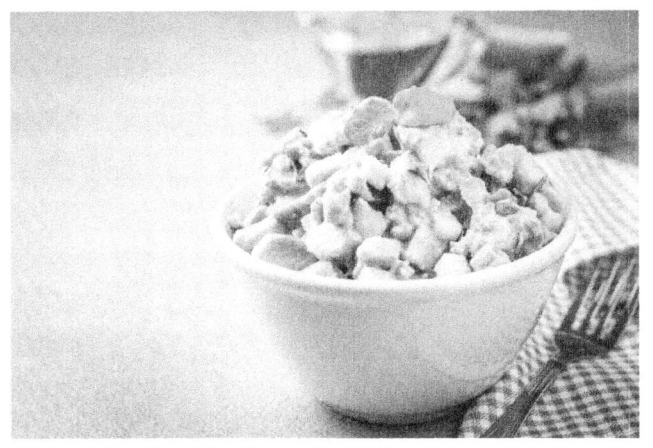

Credit: Irina Rostokina /Shutterstock.com

Macros

Prep and cook time: 10 min
Servings: 2
Fat: 36.3 g
Sodium: 2082 mg
Carbohydrates: 10.96 g
Fiber: 7.7 g
Protein: 152 g
Vitamin C: 13.7 mg
Potassium: 1966 mg
Iron: 13.5 mg
Calcium: 160 mg
Calories: 960

What you need

- 1 small cucumber diced
- ½ small avocado diced
- 1 tsp. of lemon juice
- 1 can of tuna
- 1 tbsp. of olive oil
- salad greens
- salt

Steps:

1. In a medium bowl, mix the avocado, cucumber and lemon juice.
2. Flake the tuna and mix it thoroughly with olive oil.
3. Add tuna to the cucumber and avocado mixture then add a pinch of salt.
4. Prepare the salad greens by adding lemon juice and olive oil.
5. Put the tuna salad on salad greens and serve.

AIP Soup Recipes
Beet Orange-Tarragon Soup

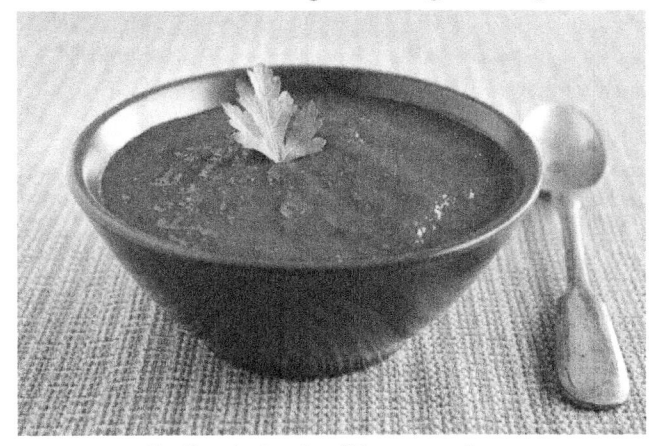

Credit: ziashusha /Shutterstock.com

Macros

Prep and cook time: 40 min
Servings: 4
Fat: 10.6 g
Sodium: 635 mg
Carbohydrates: 8.2 g
Fiber: 2.4 g
Protein: 1.8 g
Vitamin C: 5 mg
Potassium: 301 mg
Iron: 1.2 mg
Calcium: 21 mg
Calories: 129

What you need

- 3 large beetroots diced
- 2 tsp. of minced tarragon
- 2 tsp. of grated orange peels
- 2 tsp. of olive oil
- 2 tsp. of red wine vinegar
- 1 tsp. of sea salt
- ½ cup of coconut milk
- filtered water

Steps:

1. Put the diced beetroots in a medium sized pot, cover with water and allow it to boil.
2. Once boiling, reduce the heat to simmer and add the orange peels and tarragon.
3. Simmer for another 30 minutes until the beetroots are tender enough to smash using a folk.
4. Add sea salt, coconut milk, olive oil, and red wine vinegar to a blender or food processor.
5. Add the beetroots without draining the remaining water to the food processor or blender. Ensure that your food processor or blender is heat proof before adding the hot beetroots.
6. Process the ingredients on high speed until they are completely smooth.
7. Serve in small bowls and enjoy!

Garlic Scape and Asparagus Soup

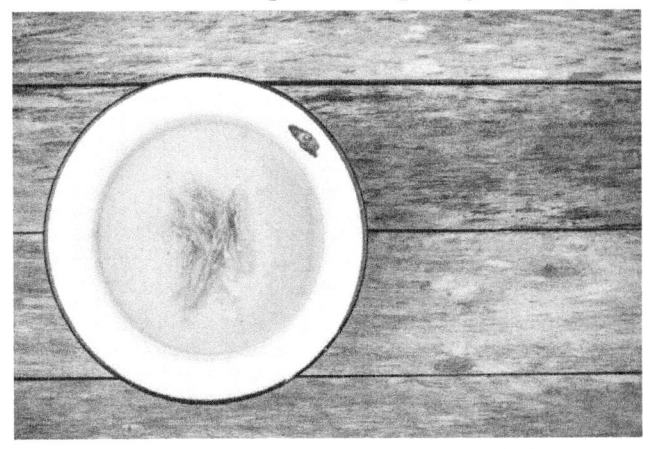

Credit: Ekaterina Kondratova /Shutterstock.com

Macros

Prep and cook time: 40 min
Servings: 4
Fat: 5 g
Sodium: 1375 mg
Carbohydrates: 7 g
Fiber: 2.6 g
Protein: 8 g
Vitamin C: 42 mg
Potassium: 537 mg
Iron: 2 mg
Calcium: 112 mg
Calories: 99

What you need

- ½ lbs. of asparagus
- 2 tsp. of olive oil
- 6 garlic scapes
- ½ lbs. of cauliflower or white sweet potatoes
- 1 tsp. of sea salt
- 4 cups of broth
- 2 cups leafy greens of your choice
- 2 tsp. of freshly pressed lemon juice

Steps:

1. In a large saucepan, boil 1 cup of water.
2. Cut the top 3 inches of the asparagus and set aside for later use.
3. Put the cut asparagus tips in a steaming basket and place over the boiling water in the saucepan.
4. Cover and allow it to steam for about 3 minutes.
5. Drain the water and put the asparagus tips in ice water and set aside.
6. In the empty saucepan, add 2 tsp. of olive oil.
7. Add roughly chopped garlic scapes and the remaining asparagus while chopped.
8. Add the sweet potatoes or cauliflower and allow it to cook for 4 minutes or until the ingredients are soft or vibrant green.
9. Add broth and salt, cover and let it simmer for 5 minutes.
10. Add the leafy greens and cook for 3 minutes or until your vegetables are soft.
11. Turn off the heat and puree the soup using an immersion blender.
12. Season with lemon juice to your liking.
13. Drain the asparagus tips from step 5, add to the soup and serve.

Creamy Artichoke Chicken Stew (Instant Pot)

Macros

Prep and cook time: 25 min
Servings: 4
Fat: 50 g
Sodium: 1475 mg
Carbohydrates: 29 g
Fiber: 11.3 g
Protein: 37.8 g
Vitamin C: 53 mg
Potassium: 1450 mg
Iron: 4.5 mg
Calcium: 168 mg
Calories: 699

What you need

- 1 small onion thinly diced
- 1 tbsp. of coconut oil
- 1 cup bone broth
- 1 cup of coconut milk
- 2 tbsp. of lemon juice
- 1 pound quartered mushrooms
- 1 can artichokes roughly chopped
- 1-pound cooked chicken - shredded
- 2 pressed garlic cloves
- 1 tbsp. of parsley
- ½ tsp. of thyme
- 1/8 tsp. of mace
- 1 tsp. salt
- ¼ cup of nutritional yeast
- 2 cups of roughly chopped spinach
- fresh parsley for garnishing

Steps:

1. Press the instant pot sauté function; add onions and coconut oil.
2. Sauté the onions for about 6 minutes until they begin to soften and brown.
3. Press the cancel/off button.
4. Add all the remaining ingredients except for the spinach and stir thoroughly.
5. Place the cover on the instant pot and ensure that the lid is well-secured.
6. Press the manual button, reduce the pressure to low and change the time to 5 minutes.
7. Let the cycle run until you hear a beeping sound then hit the cancel/off button.
8. Vent to depressurize, remove the cover and add the spinach.
9. Give a good stir, adjust seasonings and serve.

Cheeseburger Mushroom Soup

Macros

Prep and cook time: 50 minutes
Servings: 4
Fat: 28.4 g
Sodium: 1750 mg
Carbohydrates: 9.2 g
Fiber: 2.4 g
Protein: 25.3 g
Vitamin C: 5 mg
Potassium: 471 mg
Iron: 4 mg
Calcium: 99 mg
Calories: 389

What you need

- 2 tbsp. of coconut oil
- 1 lb. of grass-fed beef ground
- 1 small white onion finely diced
- 2 garlic cloves finely diced
- 2 cups of brown mushrooms thinly sliced
- 750 grams of frozen cauliflower
- 2 carrots chopped into small pieces
- 2 cups of broth
- 4 cups of water
- 1 tbsp. of dried thyme and sage each
- ½ tbsp. of turmeric
- 1 tbsp. of gelatin
- 1 tbsp. of nutritional yeast
- ½ tbsp. of balsamic vinegar
- 1 tbsp. of salt

Steps:

1. In a large stock pot, add the chopped carrots and frozen cauliflower. Add broth and water that covers the vegetables and allow it to boil.
2. Add salt, thyme, turmeric, and sage and let it simmer for about 20 minutes until the vegetables are tender soft.
3. As you wait, heat coconut oil in a skillet; add garlic, onions, and beef.
4. Cook until the beef is evenly cooked and brown.
5. Add the mushrooms and cook for another 6 minutes.
6. Once the vegetables are cooked and tender, add balsamic, nutritional yeast and gelatin to a blender and blend until smooth.
7. Add to the mushrooms and beef mixture and simmer for 5 minutes.
8. Season to taste and serve.

Veggie and Cream of Chicken Soup

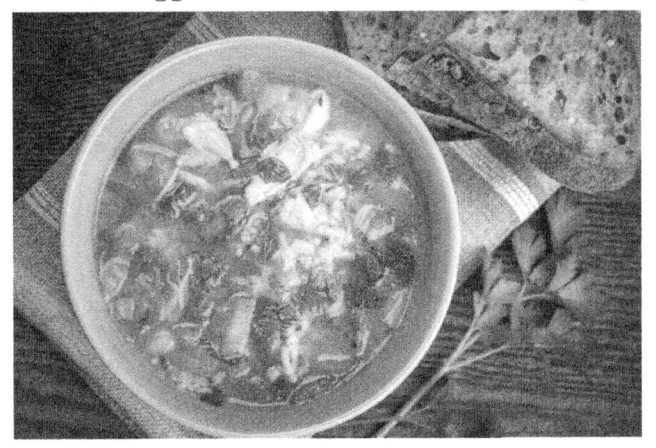

Credit: Elena Elisseeva /Shutterstock.com

Macros

Prep and cook time: 45 min
Servings: 4
Fat: 17 g
Sodium: 1150 mg
Carbohydrates: 25 g
Fiber: 4.9 g
Protein: 15.2 g
Vitamin C: 64 mg
Potassium: 871 mg
Iron: 3 mg
Calcium: 169 mg
Calories: 304

What you need

- cauliflower 4 cups
- bone broth 4 cups
- 2 cups of water
- shredded cooked chicken 2 cups
- 2 medium carrots
- 1 medium zucchini
- 8 medium brown mushrooms
- 2 tbsp. of salt
- 1 tbsp. of mixed herbs
- 1 medium lemon
- 1 cup each frozen spinach, and parsley
- 4 green spring onions

Steps:

1. In a medium sized pot, add the cauliflower, water and broth and allow them to boil until the cauliflower softens.
2. As the cauliflower cooks, thinly slice the mushrooms, dice the zucchini and carrots.
3. Add the cauliflower mixture to a blender and blend on high speed until well combined and smooth.
4. Add the mushrooms, zucchini and carrots to the cauliflower puree then add more water to cover the ingredients. Bring to simmer until the carrots soften.
5. Add the shredded chicken, frozen spinach, dried herbs, and salt.
6. Simmer for a few minutes until the spinach warms through and thaws.
7. Add the green spring onions, parsley and lemon juice.
8. Season with salt and serve.

Seafood Coconut Soup

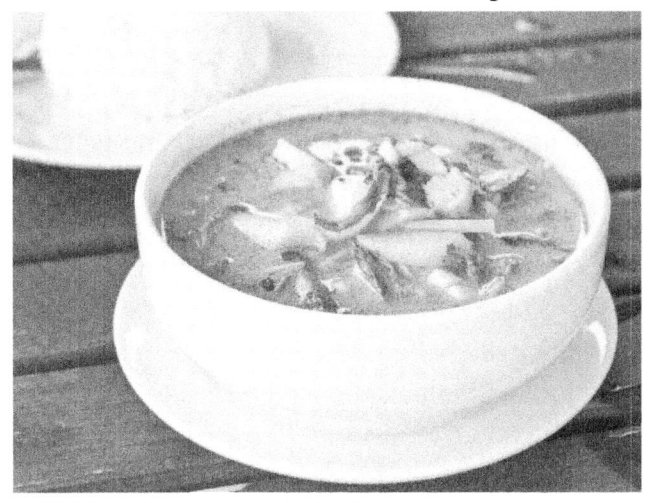

Credit: Ekkachai /Shutterstock.com

Macros

Prep and cook time: 30 min
Servings: 4
Fat: 40 g
Sodium: 262 mg
Carbohydrates: 13 g
Fiber: 2.7 g
Protein: 48 g
Vitamin C: 8 mg
Potassium: 1650 mg
Iron: 5 mg
Calcium: 39 mg
Calories: 588

What you need

- chicken stock 32 oz.
- 10 sliced mushroom buttons
- ½ cup of chopped kales
- 1 cup of chopped romaine lettuce
- 4 largely chopped tilapia filets
- 10 prawns/shrimps
- 10 mussels
- 1 cup of coconut milk
- 1 tsp. of fish sauce
- salt

Steps:

1. Add the chicken stock to a large pot and allow it to boil.
2. Add the romaine lettuce, kale, and mushrooms and boil again.
3. Add the prawns/shrimps, tilapia pieces and other seafood and boil once more.
4. The soup should cover the seafood. Add chicken stock if you need more liquid.
5. Allow it to boil for 5 minutes until the prawns/shrimps turn pink and the tilapia fillets do not appear translucent.
6. Add fish sauce, salt and coconut cream to taste. Stir gently to mix the added ingredients and be careful not to break the fish pieces.
7. Let it start boiling again, turn off the heat and serve while hot.

Apple, Carrot, Ginger and Sweet Potato Soup

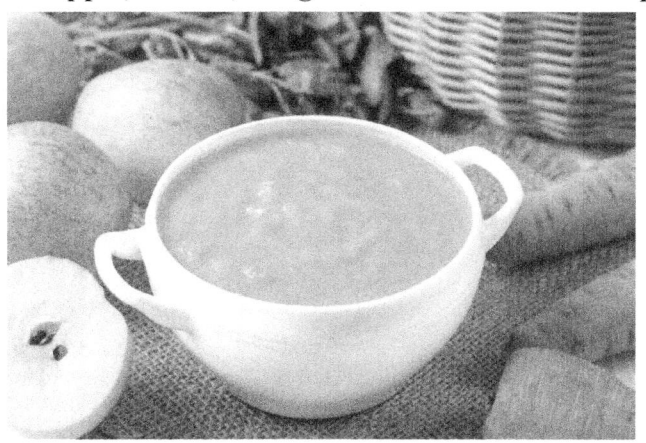

Credit: Ahanov Michael /Shutterstock.com

Macros

Prep and cook time: 45 min
Servings: 4
Fat: 17 g
Sodium: 1041 mg
Carbohydrates: 36 g
Fiber: 5.6 g
Protein: 54 g
Vitamin C: 47 mg
Potassium: 790 mg
Iron: 4 mg
Calcium: 76 mg
Calories: 521

What you need

- 3 medium sweet potatoes chopped into small pieces
- 2 medium carrots diced into small pieces
- 2 small apples chopped
- 1 large piece of peeled ginger
- 1 liter of chicken broth
- salt to taste

Steps:

1. Put everything in a large stock pot and boil for 30 minutes until all ingredients are soft.
2. Puree the mixture using an immersion blender until it smoothens.
3. Add salt to taste and serve immediately.

Chicken Ginger Soup

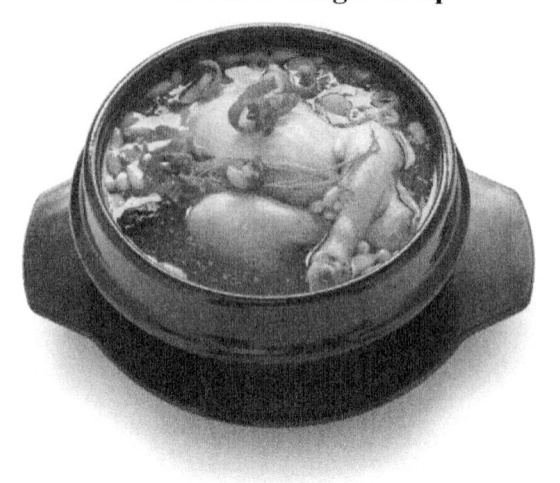

Credit: bonchan /Shutterstock.com

Macros

Prep and cook time: 60 min
Servings: 4
Fat: 6.6 g
Sodium: 486 mg
Carbohydrates: 8.7 g
Fiber: 2 g
Protein: 40 g
Vitamin C: 2 mg
Potassium: 729 mg
Iron: 3.3 mg
Calcium: 66 mg
Calories: 249

What you need

- 1.3 pounds of raw chicken
- 1 can of straw mushrooms peeled
- fresh ginger root about 4 inches
- 5 garlic cloves
- 6 cups of chicken broth
- 4 cups of water
- cilantro

Steps:

1. Transfer the water and chicken broth to a large soup pot and simmer over medium heat.
2. Cut the ginger into ½ inch discs, peel and smash the garlic.
3. Drop the garlic and ginger into the soup.
4. Allow the soup to simmer for 30 minutes to ensure all the flavors are well combined.
5. Cut the chicken into long but medium thick strips and drop them in the soup.
6. Allow the chicken to cook for 15 minutes.
7. Remove the garlic and ginger.
8. Remove the pot from heat and add in the mushrooms.
9. Garnish with cilantro and serve.

Chilled Rosemary-Blueberry Soup

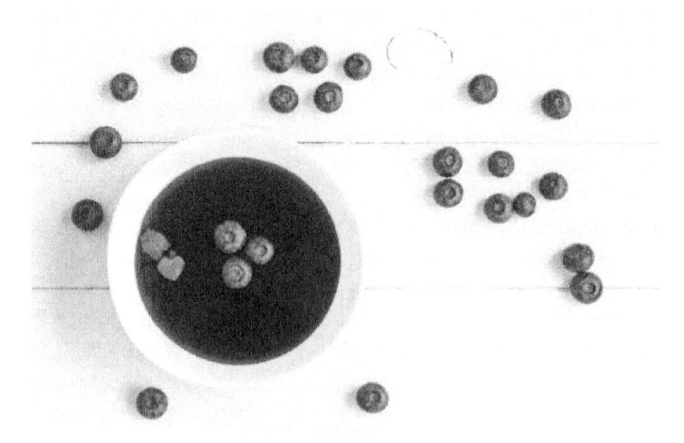

Credit: Flaffy /Shutterstock.com

Macros

Prep and cook time: 60 min
Servings: 4
Fat: 1 g
Sodium: 6 mg
Carbohydrates: 42 g
Fiber: 3.2 g
Protein: 2 g
Vitamin C: 4 mg
Potassium: 84 mg
Iron: 1 mg
Calcium: 12 mg
Calories: 171

What you need

- 3 cups of fresh blueberries
- 1 can of coconut milk
- 1/8 tsp. of minced rosemary
- ¼ tsp. of cinnamon
- 2 tsp. of apple cider vinegar
- 2 tsp. of lemon juice
- a pinch of sea salt to taste

Steps:

1. Simmer the coconut milk with apple cider vinegar, blueberries, rosemary, cinnamon, salt and lemon juice for 10 minutes.
2. The color from the blueberries will blend to form a pink/purple like soup.
3. Allow the mixture to cool at room temperature and if you are in a hurry, place it in the refrigerator for 30 minutes.
4. Pour it in a blender or food processor. Blend until you get a consistent and smooth mixture.
5. You can serve immediately or chill it. Garnish with rosemary sprig or blueberries while serving.

Shrimp and Creamy Cod Chowder

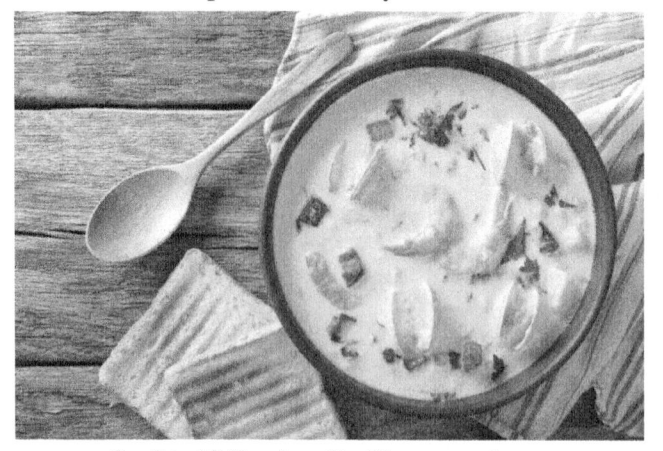

Credit: AS Food studio /Shutterstock.com

Macros

Prep and cook time: 45 min
Servings: 4
Fat: 0.4g
Sodium: 342mg
Carbohydrates: 7.7g
Fiber: 1.7g
Protein: 1.6g
Vitamin C: 5.7mg
Potassium: 327mg
Iron: 0.7mg
Calcium: 43mg
Calories: 39

What you need

- 1 lb. of cauliflower
- ¾ lbs. of parsnips
- 1 medium sized onion diced
- 4 garlic cloves
- 5 cups of seafood stock or chicken broth
- 1 tsp. of sea salt
- 1 can of coconut milk
- 1 tsp. of dill weed dried
- 1 lb. of cod fillet
- 1 lb. of deveined and peeled shrimp

Steps:

1. Chop the cauliflower roughly into florets; ensure the parsnips are peeled and trimmed.
2. Slice the parsnips and peel the garlic cloves.
3. Place a large Dutch oven over medium heat and add the parsnips, cauliflower, diced, onion, seafood stock/chicken broth, salt, and garlic.
4. Allow the stock to simmer and cook for 25 minutes or until all the vegetables are tender.
5. Turn off the heat and add coconut milk.
6. Transfer the mixture to a blender and puree until the soup gets creamy and smooth. Stir in some dried dill.
7. Place the pan back on the stove top and bring it simmer.
8. Slice the cod fillet into medium pieces and add to the soup. Also add the shrimp.
9. Cook until the code gets opaque and the shrimp turns pink; that takes about 3 minutes.
10. Serve immediately or chill overnight.

Cheese Broccoli Soup

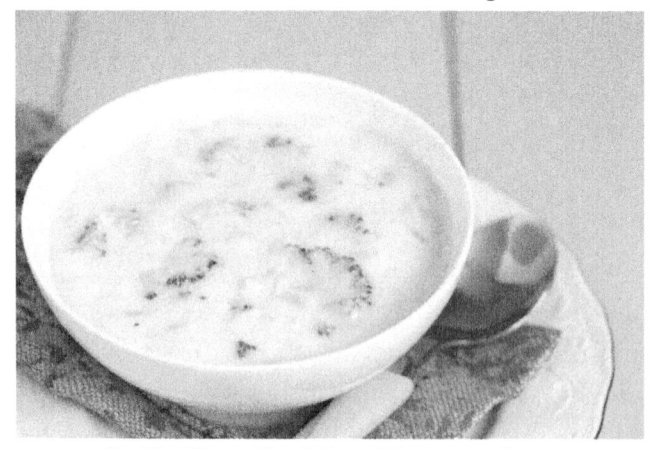

Credit: Elena Shashkina /Shutterstock.com

Macros

Prep and cook time: 30 min
Servings: 4
Fat: 65.7 g
Sodium: 2449 mg
Carbohydrates: 74.7 g
Fiber: 25 g
Protein: 80 g
Vitamin C: 15.8 mg
Potassium: 2075 mg
Iron: 10 mg
Calcium: 188 mg
Calories: 1187

What you need

- 1 can pumpkin puree
- 1 coconut milk can
- 4 cups chicken broth or stock
- 1 tbsp. of avocado oil
- ¼ cup of nutritional yeast
- 1 tbsp. of sea salt
- 1 tsp. of onion powder
- 1 tsp. of garlic powder
- 1 tsp. of dried thyme
- ½ tsp. of dried sage
- 2 tbsp. of arrowroot powder
- 6 cups of chopped broccoli

Steps:

1. In a medium sized pot, mix the coconut milk, bone broth and pumpkin puree and cook over medium heat until you get a creamy consistency.
2. Add nutritional yeast, onion powder, thyme, avocado oil, sage, sea salt, and garlic powder. Stir occasionally as they cook.
3. Once the mixture begins to boil, add the arrowroot powder (1 tbsp at a time) and whisk.
4. Add broccoli florets and cook for 7 minutes until they soften. Serve and enjoy.

Chicken Noodle Soup

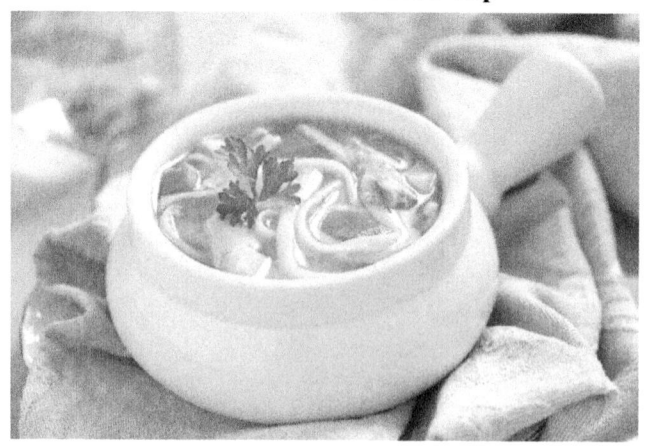

Credit: Elena Shashkina /Shutterstock.com

Macros

Prep and cook time: 30 min
Servings: 2
Fat: 52.5 g
Sodium: 1587 mg
Carbohydrates: 5.3 g
Fiber: 0.9 g
Protein: 108 g
Vitamin C: 7.4 mg
Potassium: 904 mg
Iron: 5.35 mg
Calcium: 83 mg
Calories: 955

What you need

- 3 cups of chicken broth
- 1 chopped chicken breast
- 2 tbsp. of avocado oil
- 1 chopped celery stalk
- 1 chopped green onion
- ¼ cup of finely chopped cilantro
- 1 medium peeled zucchini
- salt

Steps:

1. Place a saucepan over medium heat and add avocado oil.
2. Add the diced chicken breast and sauté until well cooked.
3. Add chicken broth and allow it to simmer.
4. Add the chopped green onions and celery.
5. Use a potato peeler, food processor or spiralizer to create zucchini noodles.
6. Add the zucchini noodles and cilantro to the saucepan.
7. Allow to simmer for a few minutes.
8. Add salt and serve while hot.

Instant Pot Fennel Beet Soup

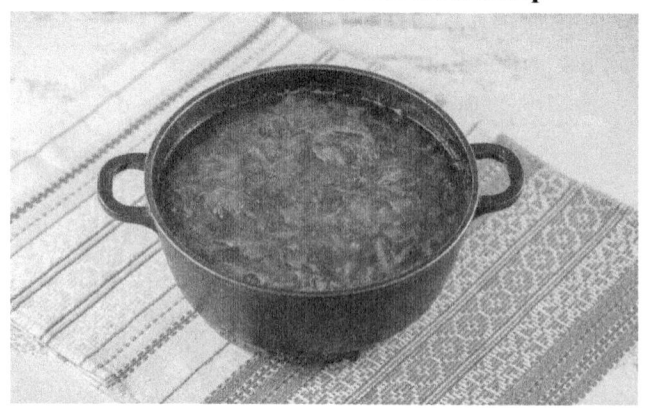

Credit: YURENIA NATALLIA /Shutterstock.com

Macros

Prep and cook time: 55 min
Servings: 4
Fat: 7 g
Sodium: 539 mg
Carbohydrates: 17.87 g
Fiber: 3.4 g
Protein: 33.6 g
Vitamin C: 7.6 mg
Potassium: 680 mg
Iron: 2.4 mg
Calcium: 50 mg
Calories: 270

What you need

- 1 tbsp. of coconut oil
- ½ chopped onion
- 1 lb. of chopped beet
- 1 chopped fennel bulb
- 3 garlic cloves halved
- 1 quarter bone or chicken broth
- 3 tbsp. of balsamic vinegar
- ¼ cup of basil leaves finely chopped
- 1 tbsp. of salt

Steps:

1. In an instant pot, put 1 tbsp. of coconut oil and melt it by pressing the sauté button.
2. Once the coconut oil is completely melted, add the chopped onions and cook for about 7 minutes until they are clear.
3. Press the off button.
4. Add all the other ingredients and give a good stir to ensure all ingredients are mixed.
5. Cover the instant pot with its lid and press the soup button.
6. Allow the soup to cook until the buzzer rings, after which you should press the off button.
7. Allow the instant pot to release pressure for about 10 minutes before opening it.
8. Pour the soup in a large food processor or blender and blend until it becomes creamy and smooth.
9. Serve immediately.

Zuppa Toscana

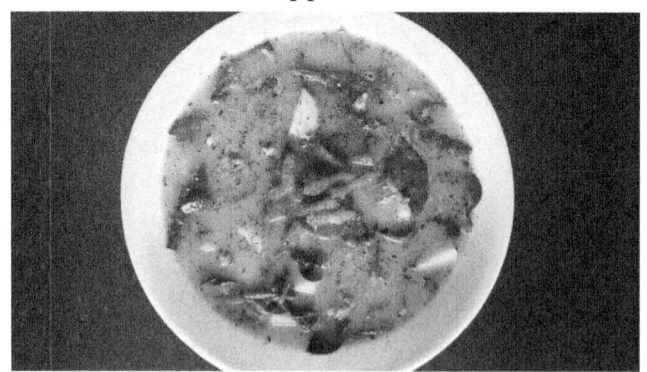

Credit: krsalomonsky /Shutterstock.com

Macros

Prep and cook time: 25 min
Servings: 4
Fat: 30 g
Sodium: 1750 mg
Carbohydrates: 39 g
Fiber: 9 g
Protein: 43 g
Vitamin C: 223 mg
Potassium: 1650 mg
Iron: 9 mg
Calcium: 311mg
Calories: 590

What you need

- 6 bacon slices
- 1 small onion finely chopped
- 1 lb. of ground beef
- 2 garlic cloves
- 4 cups of chicken broth
- 1 large chopped celeriac
- 2 cups of chopped kale
- ¼ cup of coconut milk

Steps:

1. Place a stock pot over medium heat and cook bacon pieces until they are crispy and remove them from the pan. Reserve the bacon fat.
2. Add onions to the pot and cook for about 3 minutes or until translucent.
3. Add ground beef and cook for 3 minutes, stirring regularly until it browns.
4. Add garlic and cook for another 3 minutes.
5. Add the celeriac and broth and allow them to boil then reduce the heat to simmer and cook for about 20 minutes without covering.
6. Add the coconut milk and kale then cook until the kale wilts.
5. Serve and top with the crispy bacon pieces.

Chapter Ten: Easy AIP Desserts

Strawberry White Chocolate Scones

Macros

Prep and cook time: 30 min
Servings: 4
Fat: 23 g
Sodium: 247 mg
Carbohydrates: 42 g
Fiber: 2.4 g
Protein: 2.15 g
Vitamin C: 5.4 mg
Potassium: 214 mg
Iron: 1 mg
Calcium: 59 mg
Calories: 369

What you need

- ½ cup of coconut milk
- 4 tbsp. of honey
- 3 tbsp. of coconut oil
- ½ tbsp. of vanilla extract alcohol free
- ¾ cup of coconut flour
- ¼ cup of arrowroot flour
- ½ tbsp. of baking soda
- ½ tbsp. of baking soda
- a pinch of salt
- ¼ cup of water
- 1 tbsp. of gelatin
- ¾ cup of fresh raspberries or strawberries
- ¼ cup of coconut butter chopped

Steps:

1. Start by preheating the oven at 350°F and line a medium sized cookie sheet with a parchment paper.
2. Whisk honey, coconut milk, coconut oil, and vanilla in a large bowl until smooth.
3. Add the dry ingredients gradually to the wet ingredients and whisk as you add.
4. Whisk until all the ingredients are well combined and no clumps are visible.
5. Put the water in a small pan and sprinkle the gelatin over slowly and allow it to bloom for 2 minutes.
6. Turn the heat to low for the gelatin to melt slowly then whisk until frothy to make the gelatin egg.
7. Pour the egg into the other ingredients and stir quickly.
8. Gently fold the raspberries or strawberries and coconut butter.
9. Spoon the batter in the prepared cookie sheet as rounded tablespoons.
10. Place it in the preheated oven and allow it to bake for 25 minutes or until the batter tops are browned lightly. Use a toothpick to check whether they are well cooked; if the toothpick comes out clean, you are good to go!
11. Allow it to cool completely before consuming.
12. This can be stored in the refrigerator for 1 week and 3 months in the freezer.

Swirl Cinnamon Muffins

Macros

Prep and cook time: 30 min
Servings: 4
Fat: 6.9 g
Sodium: 173 mg
Carbohydrates: 13 g
Fiber: 1.4 g
Protein: 1 g
Vitamin C: 0.5 mg
Potassium: 117 mg
Iron: 0.5 mg
Calcium: 53 mg
Calories: 116

What you need

Muffins:
- ¼ cup of coconut flour
- ¼ cup of arrowroot starch
- 2/3 cup of sifted tiger nut flour
- ½ tbsp. of baking soda
- ¼ tsp. of sea salt
- 2 tsp. of cinnamon
- 2 tsp. of coconut palm sugar or maple sugar
- 1 tsp. of apple cider vinegar
- ½ cup of coconut milk
- 6 tsp. of pure maple
- 6 tsp. of melted palm shortening
- ½ cup of apple sauce unsweetened
- 2 tsp. of gelatin
- ¼ cup of water

Swirl:
- 2 tsp. of cinnamon
- 2 tsp. of maple syrup
- 2 tsp. of melted palm shortening

Steps:

For muffins:

1. Start by preheating the oven at 350°F and line a medium sized muffin pan with a parchment paper.
2. Whisk all the dry muffin ingredients apart from the gelatin together in a large bowl.
3. In a separate medium bowl, whisk all wet muffin ingredients except for water together.
4. Add the wet ingredients to the dry ingredients and whisk as you add. Whisk this until all ingredients are well combined and smooth.
5. Put the water in a small pan and sprinkle the gelatin over slowly and allow it to bloom for 2 minutes.
6. Turn the heat to low for the gelatin to melt slowly, then whisk until frothy to make the gelatin egg.
7. Mix the gelatin egg with the muffin batter and whisk quickly.
8. Spoon the muffin batter into muffin cups ½ or ¾ way full.

Swirl:

1. Add the swirl ingredients to a small bowl and mix until well combined.
2. Pour ½ tsp. of the swirl toppings on each muffin batter. Using a toothpick, swirl the topping into the muffin batter.
3. Place in the oven and allow them to bake for 25 minutes until muffin tops are browned or until a toothpick piercing the center of the muffin comes out clean.
4. Remove the muffins from the oven and allow them to cool completely before serving.
5. These muffins can be stored in the freezer for 3 months or 5 days in the fridge.

Pomegranate Chocolate Bites

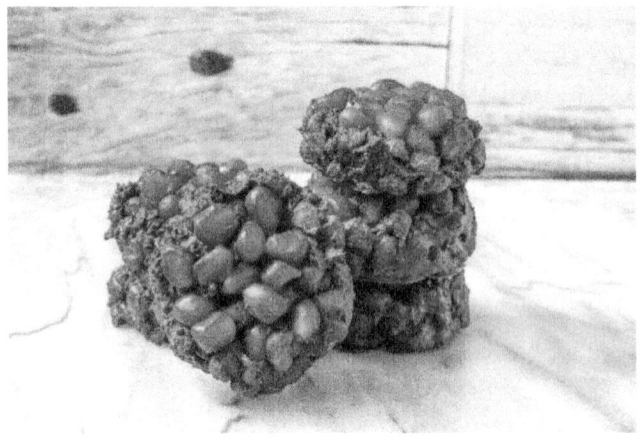

Credit: Aris Setya /Shutterstock.com

Macros

Prep and cook time: 20 min
Servings: 4
Fat: 27.7 g
Sodium: 28 mg
Carbohydrates: 32 g
Fiber: 5.3 g
Protein: 2.6 g
Vitamin C: 8 mg
Potassium: 311 mg
Iron: 1.1 mg
Calcium: 28 mg
Calories: 360

What you need

- ¼ cup of coconut oil melted
- 2 tsp. of coconut butter/manna
- 6 tsp. of honey
- ½ cup of coconut cream
- ½ tsp. of vanilla alcohol free
- 6 tsp. of carob powder roasted
- a large pomegranate

Steps:

1. Prepare the pomegranate; wash it, cut it and de-seed it. Place the seeds in a bowl and set aside.
2. Place a medium sized pan on medium heat and melt the coconut oil, coconut cream, honey, and coconut butter/manna. Keep stirring until all ingredients are melted.
3. Reduce the heat to low then add carob powder and vanilla. Whisk the ingredients until the carob dissolves completely. If the mixture starts boiling as you whisk, turn off the heat and stir a few times before turning on the heat. Remove for heat once the carob is completely smooth.
4. Add the carob mixture halfway to the silicone moulds.
5. Sprinkle some pomegranate seeds and add the remaining carob mixture.
6. Put this in the freezer for 2 hours.
7. Take from the freezer and remove the silicone moulds.
8. Freeze immediately because they melt fast at room temperature.
9. Take from the freezer just before eating.

Coconut Chocolate Peppermint Truffles

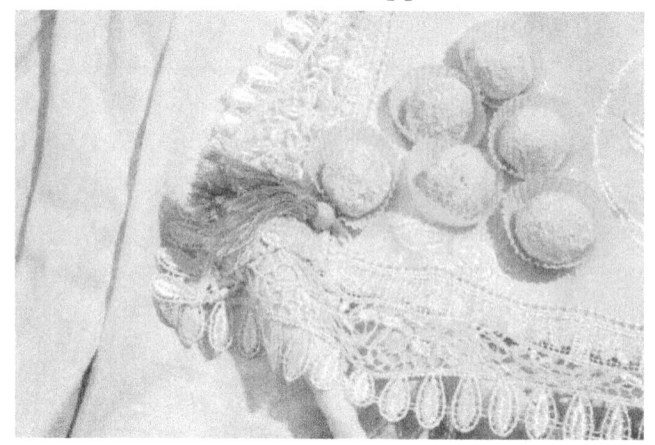

Credit: Iuliia Stepashova /Shutterstock.com

Macros

Prep and cook time: 10 minutes
Servings: 4
Fat: 10.5 g
Sodium: 51 mg
Carbohydrates: 8.7 g
Fiber: 1.4 g
Protein: 0.6 g
Vitamin C: 1.1 mg
Potassium: 150 mg
Iron: 0.22 mg
Calcium: 30 mg
Calories: 125

What you need

- 2 cups of shredded unsweetened coconut
- ¼ cup of melted coconut oil
- 4 tsp. of maple syrup
- 3 peppermint drops
- 6 tsp. of carob powder roasted
- 6 tsp. of coconut milk
- 2 tsp. of honey
- 4 tsp. of melted coconut milk

Steps:

1. Prepare a baking sheet and line it with a parchment paper.
2. Add the maple syrup, ¼ cup of coconut oil, peppermint oil, and shredded coconut to a food processor and blend until well combined and wet.
3. Squeeze the batter with your hands to form small balls.
4. Place the balls in the prepared baking sheet and freeze for 20 minutes.
5. Mix the coconut milk and carob in a small bowl. Once well combined, add melted coconut oil and honey. The coconut oil should be added 2 tsp. at a time and ensure that it is well mixed before adding more.
6. Take the coconut balls from the freezer and dip the bottoms in the chocolate. Return the balls in the baking sheet.
7. Sprinkle the remaining chocolate over the balls.
8. Return the baking sheet in the freezer for 20 minutes to allow the ingredients to set.
9. These truffles can be stored in the refrigerator for 2 weeks and 3 months in the freezer.
10. Thaw for about 5 minutes before serving.

Coconut Blueberry Popsicles

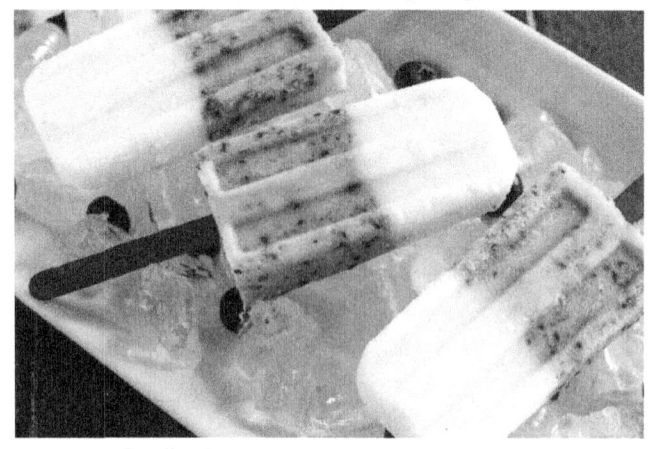

Credit: Teri Virbickis /Shutterstock.com

Macros

Prep and cook time: 10 min
Servings: 2
Fat: 1.2 g
Sodium: 15 mg
Carbohydrates: 19 g
Fiber: 1.1 g
Protein: 1.4 g
Vitamin C: 3.7 mg
Potassium: 76 mg
Iron: 0.24 mg
Calcium: 38 mg
Calories: 87

What you need

- ½ cup of blueberries
- ¼ cup of coconut milk
- 1 tsp. of raw honey
- 2 tsp. of lemon juice
- a pinch of salt

Steps:

1. Blend all ingredients together until well combined. You can use a magic bullet blender.
2. Taste and add more of the ingredients you wish.
3. Pour the mixture in ice pop molds but do not fill completely. Leave room for expansion.
4. Freeze them for at least 4 hours.
5. Once ready and well frozen, remove from the freezer and run the ice pop mould under hot water for a minute. This makes it easy to pull out the ice pops.

Sweet Potato Cookies

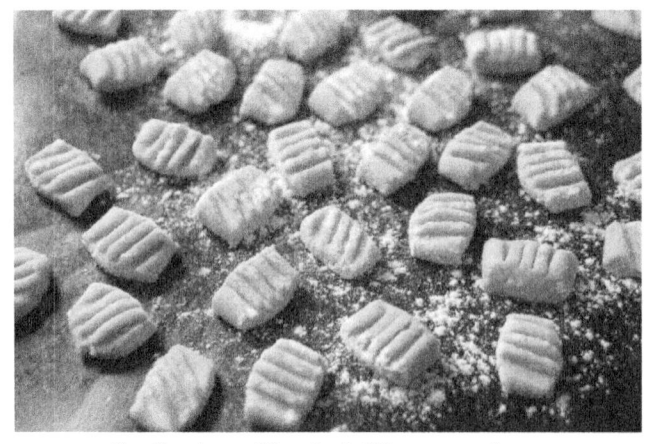

Credit: Anna Hoychuk /Shutterstock.com

Macros

Prep and cook time: 20 min
Servings: 4
Fat: 5.2 g
Sodium: 27 mg
Carbohydrates: 14.2 g
Fiber: 0.8 g
Protein: 0.7 g
Vitamin C: 6 mg
Potassium: 166 mg
Iron: 0.5 mg
Calcium: 9 mg
Calories: 101

What you need

- 200 g of grated sweet potatoes
- 6 tsp. of coconut oil
- 2 tsp. of gelatin in powder form
- 60 ml of honey
- ¾ cup of coconut flour
- 1 tsp. of baking powder

Steps:

1. Prepare the oven and preheat at 350°F.
2. Place a pan on low heat; add coconut oil and the grated sweet potatoes. Cook as you stir regularly until the sweet potato moisture dries.
3. Prepare the gelatin egg by dashing the gelatin powder over 15 ml of warm water. Once the gelatin dissolves completely, add 1 tbsp. of hot water and mix thoroughly.
4. Add honey to the sweet potatoes in the pan and cook until the moisture evaporates
5. Add the gelatin egg and combine thoroughly.
6. Turn off the heat and add ¾ cup of hot water and set the sweet potato mixture aside.
7. In a large bowl, combine the baking powder and coconut flour.
8. Add the sweet potatoes mixture to the large bowl and combine using a wooden spoon.
9. Using your hands, portion the mixture into small balls and shape them like flat cookies.
10. Place the balls in a baking tray and put it in the preheated oven. Allow it to bake for 20 minutes.
11. After 20 minutes, turn off the oven and do not open the oven door. This allows the cookies to continue cooking with the oven heat for about an hour.
12. Take the baking tray from the oven and allow the cookies to cool off completely before serving.

Stuffed Coconut Butter Dates

Macros

Prep and cook time: 10 min
Servings: 4
Fat: 46 g
Sodium: 365 mg
Carbohydrates: 13.4 g
Fiber: 1.5 g
Protein: 0.9 g
Vitamin C: 0.2 mg
Potassium: 130 mg
Iron: 0.2 mg
Calcium: 21 mg
Calories: 457

What you need

- 1 cup of coconut butter
- 10 dates pitted

Steps:

1. Slightly melt the coconut butter in a microwave. It should be soft enough to scoop with ease.
2. Slice the dates to open them up without slicing completely.
3. Stuff the dates with as much of the coconut butter as can fit in the open space and still manage to close it.
4. Enjoy!

Pumpkin Pie

Macros

Prep and cook time: 30 min
Servings: 4
Fat: 20 g
Sodium: 121 mg
Carbohydrates: 20.6 g
Fiber: 2.9 g
Protein: 8.2 g
Vitamin C: 2.3 mg
Potassium: 370 mg
Iron: 2.6 mg
Calcium: 41 mg
Calories: 274

What you need

- 1 tsp. of ground cinnamon
- 1 tsp. of ground ginger
- a pinch of ground mace
- 150 g of coconut flour
- 3 tsp. of pumpkin spice
- 5 tsp. of runny honey
- 4 tsp. of coconut oil
- 95 ml of hot water
- 2 tsp. of gelatin powder
- 300 g of pumpkin puree
- 4 tsp. of raw honey
- 80 ml of coconut milk

Steps:

For the base:

1. Prepare the oven and preheat at 355°F.
2. In a large bowl, combine a small amount of pumpkin spice with coconut flour.
3. In a small bowl, whisk the melted coconut oil, hot water and honey.
4. Add the wet mixture to the dry ingredients and mix them until you get a breadcrumb like mixture.
5. Tip the mixture into a greased pie dish and press it down to form a compact and even layer.
6. Place in the oven and let it bake for 8 minutes, turn off the oven and leave it in the oven for 10 minutes without opening the oven door.
7. Allow it cool completely.

The filling:

1. Dissolve the gelatin in hot water and set aside as you prepare the other filling ingredients.
2. Place a pan over low heat; add pumpkin spice, coconut milk, honey, and pumpkin puree. Cook for 3 minutes and you stir continuously.
3. Add the warm gelatin mixture and stir thoroughly.
4. Pour the filling over the now cooled pie dish and place in the refrigerator for a few hours to allow it to set before serving.

Marshmallows

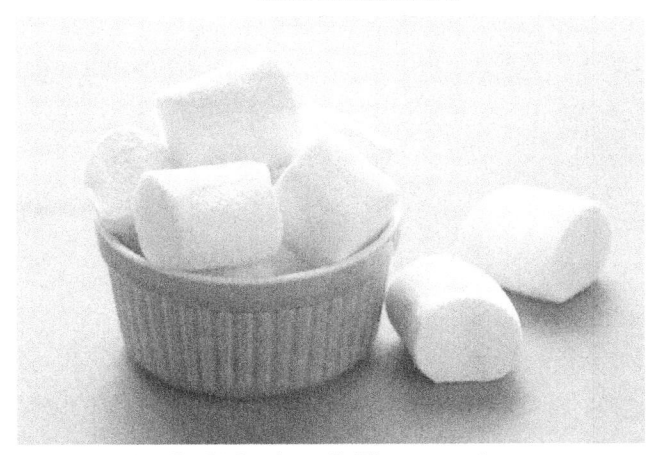

Credit: Valentina_G /Shutterstock.com

Macros

Prep and cook time: 30 min
Servings: 4
Fat: 0.01 g
Sodium: 9 mg
Carbohydrates: 15 g
Fiber: 0 g
Protein: 0.12
Vitamin C: 0.1 mg
Potassium: 6 mg
Iron: 0.1 mg
Calcium: 4 mg
Calories: 57

What you need

- ½ cup of cold water
- 6 tsp. of gelatin powder
- 75 ml of honey
- ½ cup of warm water
- avocado oil
- carob powder or arrowroot powder
- stand mixer or electric whisk

Steps:

1. Start by lining a medium size pan with a parchment paper and grease the paper with the avocado oil.
2. Sprinkle the gelatin over the ½ cup of cold water and set it aside.
3. Heat a medium size pot and add ½ cup of water and honey. Ensure the honey is well combined with the water without having to boil it too much.
4. Take the gelatin mixture and whisk it with a stand mixer or electric whisk. Start the whisking on low speed then gradually increase the speed.
5. Slowly add the honey mixture to the mixing bowl.
6. Continue whisking for another 10 minutes until the mixture is creamy and white.
7. Whisk again for 10 minutes until the mixture becomes very thick and resembles marshmallow fluff.
8. Pour the resulting mixture in the earlier prepared container and refrigerate for a few hours to allow the gelatin to set.
9. Remove from the fridge and dust it with carob powder or arrowroot powder.
10. Cut to your desired shape using a greased knife and serve.

Raw Brownie Bites

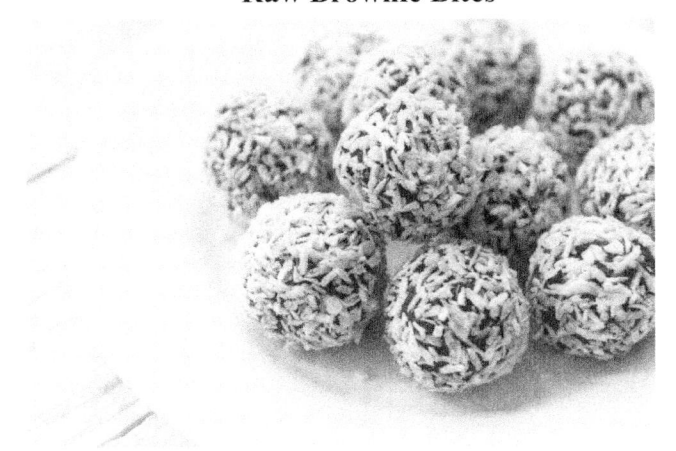

Credit: Vladyslav Rasulov /Shutterstock.com

Macros

Prep and cook time: 30 min
Servings: 5
Fat: 5.3 g
Sodium: 10 mg
Carbohydrates: 50 g
Fiber: 4.9 g
Protein: 1.4 g
Vitamin C: 0.4 mg
Potassium: 363 mg
Iron: 0.6 mg
Calcium: 29 mg
Calories: 190

What you need

- 400 g of soft dates
- 6 tsp. of carob powder
- 6 tsp. of melted coconut oil
- ¼ cup of shredded and unsweetened coconut

Steps:

1. Put the melted coconut oil, carob powder, and dates in a mini food processor and blend until well combined.
2. Transfer the mixture to a lined tray and use a metal spoon to flatten it to form a large square about ¾ inches thick.
3. Sprinkle the shredded coconut and press it gently over the surface with clean hands.
4. Refrigerate for 20 minutes then slice into squares of about 1-inch thickness.
5. Store them in the fridge while covered.

Chapter Eleven: Easy AIP Snacks

Zucchini Fries

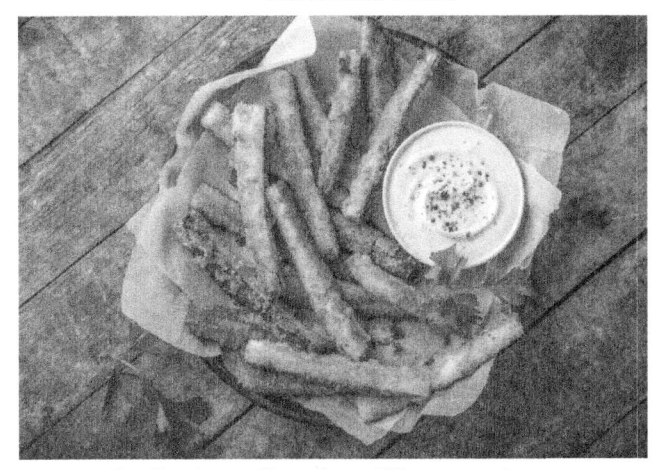

Credit: Anna Shepulova /Shutterstock.com

Macros

Prep and cook time: 55 min
Servings: 4
Fat: 21.3 g
Sodium: 447 mg
Carbohydrates: 0.53 g
Fiber: 0.1 g
Protein: 6.4 g
Vitamin C: 3.4 mg
Potassium: 145 mg
Iron: 0.6 mg
Calcium: 5 mg
Calories: 219

What you need

- 3 large zucchinis
- ¼ cup of olive oil
- 1 pack of pork rinds 3 oz.

Steps:

1. Prepare two baking trays and line each with a parchment paper.
2. Preheat the oven at 400°F.
3. Slice the zucchinis into 1/3-inch fry shape pieces.
4. Use a food processor to finely grind the pork rinds and pour them in a baking dish.
5. Put olive oil and zucchinis in a zip top bag and shake well to coat zucchini with oil.
6. Dredge the zucchinis with pork rinds and put them on the trays as a single layer
7. Place in the oven and allow them to bake for about 40 minutes until they are crispy and brown.

Fried Apricot Tuna Bites

Macros

Prep and cook time: 20 min
Servings: 4
Fat: 14.5 g
Sodium: 1947 mg
Carbohydrates: 14 g
Fiber: 1.3 g
Protein: 150 g
Vitamin C: 2.5 mg
Potassium: 1488 mg
Iron: 13.4 mg
Calcium: 144 mg
Calories: 793

What you need

- 5 medium apricots sliced in half
- 2 cans of flaked tuna
- 2 tbsp. of thyme leaves
- 2 tbsp. of olive oil
- coconut oil
- 5 halved blueberries
- salt

Steps:

1. Add a few teaspoons of coconut oil in a frying pan and fry the apricots until they are lightly browned.
2. In a medium bowl, combine the thyme leaves, tuna, salt and olive oil.
3. Using a spoon, pile the tuna mixture mounds on the apricots.
4. Top the tuna apricots with half blueberries.

Coconut and Banana Balls

Macros

Prep and cook time: 25 min
Servings: 4
Fat: 6 g
Sodium: 133 mg
Carbohydrates: 24.7 g
Fiber: 3 g
Protein: 1.5 g
Vitamin C: 3.7 mg
Potassium: 542 mg
Iron: 0.53 mg
Calcium: 28 mg
Calories: 150

What you need

- 1 medium banana
- 2 cups of shredded coconut unsweetened
- 1 tbsp. of raw honey
- 2 tbsp. of melted coconut oil
- 1 tsp. of vanilla extract alcohol free version
- carob powder
- a pinch of salt

Steps:

1. If you like to serve balls warm, preheat the oven at 250°F.
2. In a large bowl, mix all the ingredients together to make dough.
3. Form small balls about an inch in diameter using your hands.
4. Bake or refrigerate for 15 minutes.

Avocado Zucchini Burgers

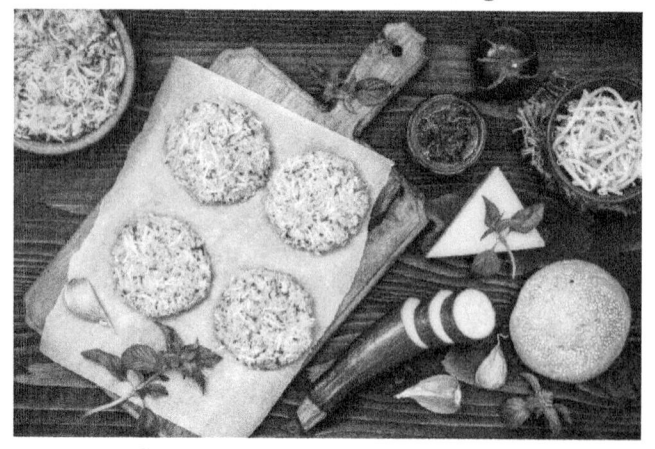

Credit: zarzamora /Shutterstock.com

Macros

Prep and cook time: 25 min
Servings: 2
Fat: 30 g
Sodium: 239 mg
Carbohydrates: 2.4 g
Fiber: 1.8 g
Protein: 30.9 g
Vitamin C: 5.2 mg
Potassium: 499 mg
Iron: 3.5 mg
Calcium: 21 mg
Calories: 405

What you need

- 1 large zucchini chopped
- ½ pound of ground beef
- ¼ avocado sliced
- 2 tbsp. of avocado or olive oil
- 1 tbsp. of salt

Steps:

1. Preheat the oven to 400°F.
2. Grease the baking tray with either avocado oil or olive oil and sprinkle salt.
3. Put the zucchini slices on the baking tray.
4. Using your hands, form small balls of ground beef and press to make patties.
5. Place the patties on the baking tray as well.
6. Put the baking tray in the preheated oven and bake for about 15 minutes.
7. Slice the avocado into small pieces.
8. Using the zucchini as buns, put the mini burgers together and add a slice of avocado on each burger.

Savory and Sweet Fried Plantains

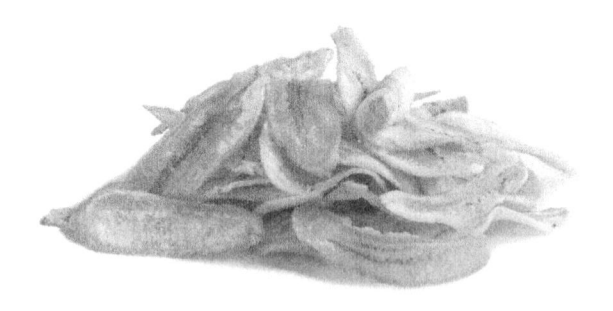

Credit: keeplight /Shutterstock.com

Macros

Prep and cook time: 20 min
Servings: 3
Fat: 18 g
Sodium: 4 mg
Carbohydrates: 27.56 g
Fiber: 2.3 g
Protein: 1.1 g
Potassium: 342 mg
Iron: 0.45 mg
Calcium: 7 mg
Calories: 273

What you need

Savory plantains:
- 1 medium and yellow plantain
- 1 tbsp. of duck fat
- ¼ tsp. of garlic powder
- a pinch of sea salt

Sweet plantains:
- 1 medium and yellow plantain
- 1 tbsp. of coconut oil
- ¼ tsp. of cinnamon
- 1 tbsp. of coconut butter

Steps:

1. Peel and slice the plantains.
2. Place two skillets on medium heat; add coconut oil in one and epic duck fat in the other.
3. Fry the plantains for about 3 minutes each side and be keen not to burn them.
4. Remove the plantain from the heat once browned and place on a paper towel lined tray. Allow the plantains to cool then transfer them to separate bowls.
5. In one bowl, drizzle coconut butter and cinnamon and in the other, sprinkle sea salt and garlic powder.
6. Serve while still warm.

Blueberry Pie Bites

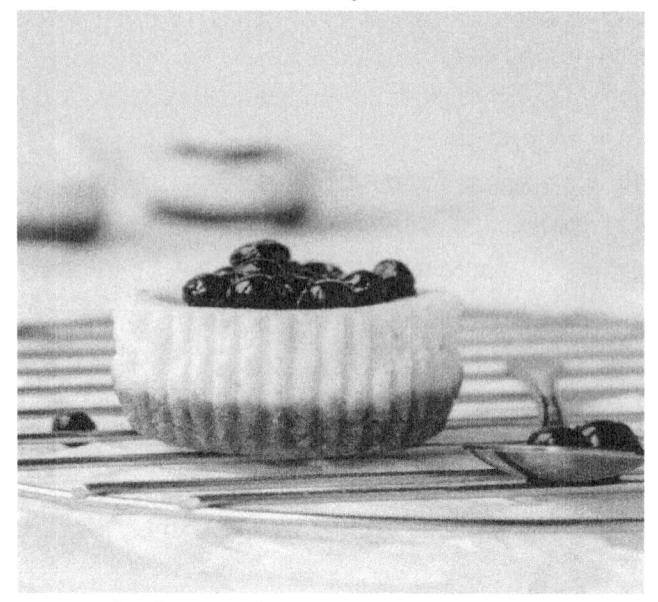

Credit: Natallia Yeupak /Shutterstock.com

Macros

Prep and cook time: 15 min
Servings: 4
Fat: 23.7 g
Sodium: 171 mg
Carbohydrates: 12.88 g
Fiber: 2 g
Protein: 0.65 g
Vitamin C: 1.4 mg
Potassium: 61 mg
Iron: 0.24 mg
Calcium: 12 mg
Calories: 258

What you need

- 2 cups of frozen or fresh blueberries
- 1 tbsp. of honey
- 1 tsp. of lemon juice
- ½ tsp. of cinnamon
- ½ cup of coconut butter
- 1 tbsp. of coconut oil
- ½ cup of shredded and unsweetened coconut flakes
- sea salt to taste

Steps:

1. Place a sauce pan over medium heat and simmer the berries with lemon juice for about 10 minutes.
2. Add a pinch of sea salt and cinnamon and stir. Transfer to a bowl and set aside.
3. Rinse the sauce pan and place back on low heat.
4. Melt the coconut butter then add the coconut shreds, coconut oil and salt.
5. Put the resulting coconut butter in muffin molds and place in the fridge for at least 20 minutes or until completely solid.
6. Pour the blueberries on the coconut base evenly and refrigerate for 2 hours or overnight for the flavors to develop.
7. Top it with whipped coconut cream, lemon zest or cinnamon.

Baked Cinnamon Banana Chips

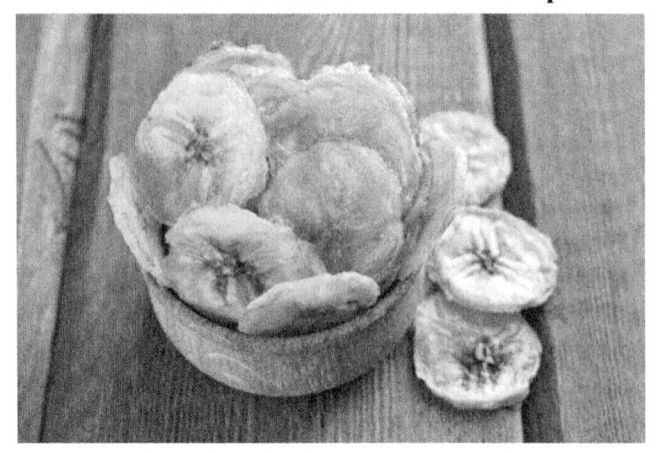

Credit: Tatiana Volgutova/Shutterstock.com

Macros

Prep and cook time: 5 minutes
Servings: 3
Fat: 1.8 g
Sodium: 3 mg
Carbohydrates: 88 g
Fiber: 9.9 g
Protein: 3.9 g
Vitamin C: 7 mg
Potassium: 1491 mg
Iron: 1.15 mg
Calcium: 22 mg
Calories: 346

What you need

- 3 tbsp. of avocado oil or coconut oil
- 3 tsp. of cinnamon
- 3 cups of unsweetened banana chips
- 2 tbsp. of maple syrup

Steps:

1. Heat the oven to 350°F.
2. Melt the cinnamon, maple syrup, and oil together.
3. Put the unsweetened banana chips in a bowl and pour the oil mixture on top.
4. Stir until the banana chips are evenly coated with the oil mixture.
5. Line a baking tray with parchment paper and spread the banana chips in one layer.
6. Place in the oven and allow the banana chips to bake for 8 minutes.
7. Allow the banana chips to cool off before indulging.
8. Store in an airtight container.

Apple Salsa

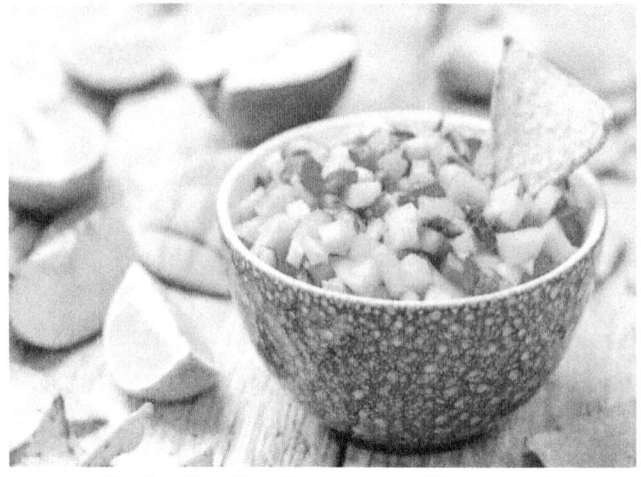

Credit: Nataliya Arzamasova /Shutterstock.com

Macros

Prep and cook time: 15 min
Servings: 2
Fat: 0.16 g
Sodium: 4 mg
Carbohydrates: 9.83 g
Fiber: 1.9 g
Protein: 0.58 g
Vitamin C: 4.7 mg
Potassium: 150 mg
Iron: 0.3 mg
Calcium: 13 mg
Calories: 42

What you need

- 2 medium apples peeled and diced
- ½ cucumber peeled and diced
- 1 large shallot diced
- ¼ cup of chopped cilantro
- 2 tbsp. of apple cider vinegar
- salt

Steps:

1. Add all the ingredients in a medium size bowl and combine thoroughly.
2. Serve and enjoy!

Strawberry Salsa

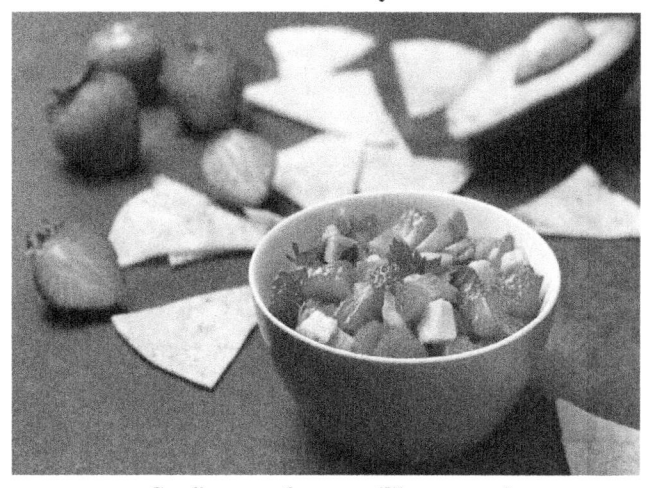

Credit: natashamam /Shutterstock.com

Macros

Prep and cook time: 20 min
Servings: 2
Fat: 0.29 g
Sodium: 4 mg
Carbohydrates: 12.58 g
Fiber: 4.7 g
Protein: 1.04 g
Vitamin C: 60.3 mg
Potassium: 231 mg
Iron: 0.72 mg
Calcium: 22 mg
Calories: 5

What you need

- 1 cup of diced strawberries
- 1 cup of diced jicama
- 1 minced shallot
- 2 tbsp. of chopped cilantro
- 2 tbsp. of fresh lime juice or white vinegar
- salt

Steps:

1. Put all the ingredients in a large bowl and stir until well combined.
2. Serve immediately.

Shrimp Ceviche

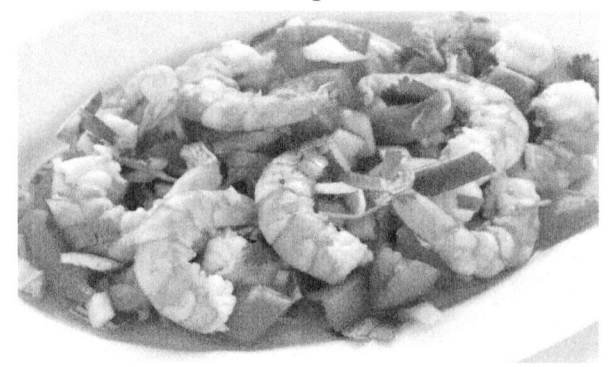

Credit: bonchan /Shutterstock.com

Macros

Prep and cook time: 30 min
Servings: 4
Fat: 10 g
Sodium: 4350 mg
Carbohydrates: 14 g
Fiber: 6 g
Protein: 24 g
Vitamin C: 31 mg
Potassium: 566 mg
Iron: 5 mg
Calcium: 198 mg
Calories: 232

What you need

- 1 lb. of shrimp
- 2 tbsp. of salt
- ½ cup of lime juice
- ¼ cup of lemon juice
- 1 large red onion chopped finely
- 1 cup of chopped cilantro
- 1 medium cucumber diced
- 2 avocados cut into chunks

Steps:

1. Put the shrimp in a large bowl.
2. Sprinkle 2 tbsp. of salt then add the lemon and lime juices over the shrimp.
3. Add cilantro, cucumber, and cilantro and toss.
4. Refrigerate for 30 minutes to allow the ingredients to marinate.
5. Add the avocado chunks and serve.

STEP 5:
EMBRACE CONTINUOUS LEARNING ABOUT AIP DIET

Chapter Twelve: Frequently Asked Questions

Why the AIP Diet?

Some histamine or high inflammatory foods are attributed to a leaky gut that in turn triggers the development of autoimmune diseases. Such foods include gluten, grains, alcohol, processed and artificial sugars, nightshades, vegetable oils, eggs, dairy products and beans. The AIP diet plays a major role in repairing the leaky gut and alleviating autoimmune diseases by eliminating foods that trigger inflammation. The AIP diet emphasizes the consumption of anti-inflammatory and gut loving foods that nourish the gut and help the body to heal and regenerate.

What Does it Mean When an Autoimmune Disease is in Remission?

Remission is defined as the disappearance of a disease as a result of treatment or diet and lifestyle change. This means that you will not experience any symptoms related to the autoimmune disease as a result of treatment and in this case, diet and lifestyle change. Complete remission occurs when the disease completely disappears and the symptoms do not re-occur. Therefore, when someone says that they are in remission, they mean that their symptoms are reduced drastically and they are able to lead a somewhat normal lifestyle.

How Do You Know Whether to Eliminate Foods for 30, 60, or 90 Days?

Though it can be challenging to know exactly how long you should adhere to the elimination diet, it is always advisable to start the reintroduction phase once you feel fully recovered. On the other hand, if you do not feel stressed out about following the AIP diet, and you are enjoying your food options, it would be wise to go on for another month or two without introducing any new foods. However, if you feel stressed out about adhering to the AIP diet, it would be advisable to start the food reintroduction stage as soon as you feel ready because this may reduce your stress.

Why is it Important to Wait 3 to 5 Days Between Food Reintroductions?

The AIP diet eliminates certain foods that cause inflammatory symptoms and the leaky gut. Since people react differently to different foods, the reintroduction stage helps you identify foods that you can tolerate and in what amounts. Therefore, it is important to wait 3 to 5 days after reintroducing a food in order to observe your body's reaction to the food. It is possible to experience delayed reactions to certain foods. For instance, if you reintroduce an egg yolk and then reintroduce macadamia after two days and experience a headache a day after, it would be hard to determine whether the headache resulted from the macadamia or the egg yolk reintroduction.

Beyond AIP Diet, is There Something Else You Should Do?

The AIP diet goes beyond the foods you consume and eliminate. Diet in Latin means a way of life. Therefore, for a person suffering from an autoimmune disease, you must adopt an anti-inflammatory lifestyle. This entails regular physical activity and stress mitigation. Considering the fact that most of the autoimmune diseases and conditions result from poor diet, lack of physical exercise and stress, addressing these factors head on is important. It not only helps to alleviate the underlying autoimmune disease symptoms but it also plays a major role in preventing the development of other lifestyle conditions such as diabetes and hypertension.

What is the Importance of Having a Shopping List?

The AIP diet focuses on ensuring that your body functions optimally in order to alleviate symptoms associated with autoimmune diseases. Therefore, it is paramount to adhere to the AIP diet in order to ensure that you not only alleviate symptoms but also achieve full recovery in the long run. This explains why it is important to have a detailed shopping list to ensure that you do not fail to buy an important ingredient. This is especially true if you restock home and kitchen supplies monthly, bi-weekly or weekly. For instance, if you will be following the 14-days meal plan as explained in this book, it is important that you have all the required kitchen supplies that can sustain you for at least one week. This will ensure that you follow the 14-day meal plan to the letter without having excuses to use non-compliant ingredients or spices to prepare your meals.

Is it Possible to Personalize Future Eating Habits?

The aim of the AIP diet is to not only foster the healing of underlying autoimmune diseases such as Hashimoto's, but also to help you lead a healthier lifestyle. This entails changing your eating habits by eliminating the consumption of fast foods, processed sugars and processed foods as well as inflammation causing foods. Moreover, the re-introduction stage allows each person to know what types of foods and spices their bodies can and cannot handle and in what quantities. This way, you are able to personalize your future eating habits by incorporating the foods your body can tolerate and in the right quantities, and by eliminating the foods that trigger inflammation and recurrence of autoimmune diseases.

Ways to Save Money While on AIP Diet

The current American food culture has made most people too lazy to even fix the quickest meal because there is always a convenient fast food option. However, in order to save money and time while on the AIP diet, it is advisable to cook in bulk and if you have busy weekdays, it is advisable to cook during the weekends and refrigerate the food. This way, you will always have something healthy and AIP compliant to eat even when you are tired or lack the time to fix a healthy meal. Additionally, it is advisable to buy your supplies in bulk for discounts or buy products that are on offer in bulk.

What if You Do Not See an Improvement?

As discussed in the previous chapters, AIP diet works differently among different people. Therefore, one person can begin experiencing change after just two weeks while another may require at least a month or more. Therefore, if you do not see any improvement, it is advisable to continue with the diet a little longer and re-evaluate your eating and lifestyle habits to ensure that you are doing everything as required as per the AIP diet guidelines. However, patience is important while on diet. Keep tabs of the small improvements because they motivate you to work harder at achieving the ultimate improvement and relieve from autoimmune diseases. A healthy and positive mindset sets you up for success.

Tips and Tricks for AIP Diet Success

Eat nutrient dense and anti-inflammatory foods. Nutrient density is a core component of the AIP diet because each body system requires a collection of nutrients to function effectively and ward off opportunistic infections and diseases. Therefore, the secret to ensuring AIP diet success is consuming nutrient rich foods. Some of the key nutrients include zinc, vitamin A and vitamin D. You can achieve this by consuming a wide variety of fruits and vegetables throughout the day. Even when you do not have complete meals, ensure that you have substantial portions of fruits and vegetables.

Helpful Resources

The Paleo Mom is an award-winning website that is dedicated to explaining how diet and lifestyle choices impact health and immunity and trigger autoimmune diseases. Hence, it is a great resource for people who wish to make positive and permanent diet and lifestyle changes towards better health. The website is owned and managed by Dr. Sarah Ballantyne, PhD. You will find AIP and Paleo diet tips to help you get through the different lifestyle change stages. Here is a link to the website https://www.thepaleomom.com/.

Unbounded wellness is a website by Michelle Hoover. Michelle, who managed to suppress Hashimoto's and digestive issues by adhering to the AIP diet, started the website as a platform to share tips and ideas of how a person can enjoy healthy foods and build a sustainable lifestyle. The website offers a wide range of lifestyle strategies suited for different people as well as diverse recipes. Here is a link https://unboundwellness.com/.

Autoimmune wellness is a blog owned and run by two incredible women; Angie and Mickey. Angie and Mickey recovered from health crisis that had been triggered by autoimmune diseases. As a result, they opted to start blogging as a way to create awareness about AIP diet by sharing personal experiences on how they relied on the autoimmune protocol diet to regain full body health and suppress autoimmune diseases. The website is dedicated to helping all autoimmune disease sufferers worldwide who are ready to start a new and unique healing journey. Here is a link to the blog https://autoimmunewellness.com/.

Strict AIP – Elimination, Reintroduction, Advice and Support is a Facebook group created to connect people who are dedicated to living on the AIP diet. It is a platform where people can share their daily challenges and wins as a way of encouraging each other especially during the elimination stage. Also, members post recipe ideas and tips to make the AIP diet much easier, fun and manageable. Visit the group via the following link https://www.facebook.com/groups/1765317403798718/.

Healing autoimmune is a website that was started by a lady known as Louise, after she managed to heal angioedema through adopting the AIP diet and lifestyle. She started the website to provide people who suffer from different autoimmune diseases with support and advice through their AIP healing journey. The website offers a wide range of AIP resources and numerous easy fix AIP recipes. Learn more here https://healingautoimmune.com/.

Final Words

Autoimmune diseases are an epidemic in society that affects millions of people in America alone. Though genetic predisposition increases the risk of developing autoimmune diseases, a person's lifestyle, diet and environment play a major role in mitigating the development of such conditions. As you may have learned from this book, certain dietary factors are key contributors to the development of autoimmune diseases.

This means that autoimmune diseases such as Hashimoto's and hypothyroidism are directly related to the lifestyle and food choices we make. As such, it is possible to manage and reverse the effects of autoimmune diseases by simply changing your diet and making well informed choices about stress, physical activity and sleep.

Foods are classified as having two main constituents; they can either promote health or undermine it. Health promoting foods offer tons of beneficial constituents and zero to minimal constituents that undermine your health. These are referred to as super foods, and they include most vegetables, seafood and organic meats. Some foods are considered as obvious to avoid because they do not have significant health promoting constituents and tend to contain problematic compounds. They include most soy products, peanuts and grains containing gluten.

However, most foods fall in between the two food extremes. For instance, tomatoes contain good nutrients but they also contain compounds that stimulate the immune system to attack itself. In light of this, the AIP diet emphasizes nutrient dense foods that not only give the body the nutrients it requires to remain healthy, but they also aid in healing the leaky gut and alleviating the symptoms of Hashimoto's and hypothyroidism.

This book has offered over 100 AIP compliant recipes to help you make this change of diet easy and convenient. Use the handy grocery lists to ensure you have AIP compliant ingredients in the house. Switching to the AIP diet is not expensive, especially if you shop with your list, and try to buy in bulk.

To succeed at the AIP diet, you just need proper planning and commitment towards living the AIP lifestyle. Have a meal plan that you adhere to strictly and cook extra food when you have the time. For instance, if you are free on Sundays, you can cook a week's worth of food and store it in the refrigerator. This eliminates your chances of consuming foods that may not be AIP compliant since you will have a quick meal ready and available anytime you need to eat.

The AIP diet requires an alteration of your lifestyle as well as changing the way you eat. In order to attain the desired results within the shortest time possible, and ensure that you increase your overall health, you must look at lifestyle factors. As you purposefully change your diet, also plan on adopting a healthier lifestyle that emphasizes less stress, more physical activities and enough sleep.

In as much as adhering to an AIP diet is proven to improve and alleviate autoimmune disease symptoms, it is important to maintain close contacts with your doctor. Always go in for check-ups and discuss any symptom changes with your physician.

What is the most important for you to understand is that improving your health begins with you! Make smart food choices! Choose the AIP diet and lifestyle to help you improve your health and your resilience to autoimmune diseases like Hashimoto's and hypothyroidism.

Dr. Wendy Sherman

Resources

Ajjan, Ramzi A., and Anthony P. Weetman. "The pathogenesis of Hashimoto's thyroiditis: further developments in our understanding." *Hormone and Metabolic Research* 47, no. 10 (2015): 702-710.

Akamizu, Takashi, and Nobuyuki Amino. "Hashimoto's thyroiditis." In *Endotext [Internet]*. MDText. com, Inc., 2017.

Alt, Angie. Beet orange-tarragon soup. https://autoimmunewellness.com/beetsoup/

Alt, Angie. Garlic and lime pan fried white fish. https://autoimmunewellness.com/angie-september-recipe/

Alt, Angie. Sheet Pan Lemon-Herb Lamb & Veggies. https://autoimmunewellness.com/sheet-pan-lemon-herb-lamb-and-veggies/

Anne Marie. Nomato sauce. https://grassfedsalsa.com/blog/nomato-sauce-aip-marinara/

Ashley, Meagen. Coconut chocolate peppermint truffles. https://www.itsallaboutaip.com/chocolate-peppermint-coconut-truffles-aip-paleo/

Ashley, Meagen. Pomegranate chocolate bites. https://www.itsallaboutaip.com/682/

Ashley, Meagen. Strawberry white chocolate scones. https://www.itsallaboutaip.com/white-chocolate-strawberry-scones-aip-paleo/

Ashley, Meagen. Swirl cinnamon muffins. https://www.itsallaboutaip.com/cinnamon-swirl-muffins/

Barrington, Kate. *The Hashimoto's Thyroiditis Healing Diet: A Complete Program for Eating Smart, Reversing Symptoms and Feeling Great.* Ulysses Press, 2016.

Bethany Tapp, Zucchini fries. https://www.thepaleomom.com/zucchini-fries-bethany-tapp/

Bryant, Rachael. Green onion and cilantro pork burgers. https://meatified.com/cilantro-pork-burgers/

Bryant, Rachael. Shrimp and creamy cod chowder. https://meatified.com/creamy-cod-shrimp-chowder/

Bryant, Rachel. Crunchy Cinnamon Baked Banana Chips. https://meatified.com/crunchy-cinnamon-banana-chips/

Chen, Beth. AIP hot pot. https://bonaippetit.com/aip-hot-pot/

Chen, Beth. Apple salsa. https://bonaippetit.com/apple-salsa/

Chen, Beth. Cauliflower rice pilaf with baked fish. https://bonaippetit.com/baked-fish-with-cauliflower-rice-pilaf-sheet-pan-meal/

Chen, Beth. Mushroom and turkey lettuce wrap. https://bonaippetit.com/turkey-and-mushroom-lettuce-wraps/

Chen, Beth. Sheet pan steak. https://bonaippetit.com/sheet-pan-steak-dinner/

Chen, Beth. Shrimp ceviche. https://bonaippetit.com/aip-shrimp-ceviche/

Chen, Beth. Strawberry salsa. https://bonaippetit.com/strawberry-salsa/

Chistiakov, Dimitry A. "Immunogenetics of Hashimoto's thyroiditis." *Journal of autoimmune diseases* 2, no. 1 (2005): 1.

Darwin, Bethany. Cheeseburger mushroom soup. http://adventuresinpartaking.com/2015/11/mushroom-cheeseburger-soup-aip-paleo-whole30-updated-march-2017/

Darwin, Bethany. Cream of chicken and veggie soup (AIP, Paleo, whole 30, dairy free). http://adventuresinpartaking.com/2015/08/cream-of-chicken-and-veggie-soup-aip-paleo-whole-30-dairy-free/#tasty-recipes-2306

Darwin, Bethany. Tuna bites. http://adventuresinpartaking.com/2015/09/tuna-bites-aip-paleo-whole30/

Dorman, Deanna. Sweet potato skins. https://blog.paleohacks.com/sweet-potato-skins/#

Elte, J. W., Aart H. Mudde, and AC Nieuwenhuijzen Kruseman. "Subclinical thyroid disease." *Postgraduate medical journal* 72, no. 845 (1996): 141-146.

Emmitt, Bre'anna. Rosemary garlic breadsticks. https://www.thepaleomom.com/guest-post-breanna-emmitt-garlic-rosemary-breadsticks-autoimmune-protocol-friendly/

Feindel, Christina. Squash browns. https://autoimmunewellness.com/squashbrowns/

Feindel, Christina. Zuppa Toscana. https://autoimmunewellness.com/zuppa-toscana/

Haber, Alaena. Blueberry pie bites. https://grazedandenthused.com/no-bake-blueberry-pie-energy-bites-aip-friendly/

Hartman, Jaime. Garlic scape and asparagus soup. https://gutsybynature.com/2019/05/28/asparagus-garlic-scape-soup-aip-scd/

Hendon, Louise. AIP Beef Stew Recipe with Cauliflower Mash. https://healingautoimmune.com/aip-beef-stew-recipe-cauliflower-mash

Hendon, Louise. AIP ceviche. https://healingautoimmune.com/aip-ceviche-recipe

Healy, Hannah. AIP chicken finger. https://healyeatsreal.com/chicken-finger-recipe/

Hendon, Louise. AIP raw brownie bites recipe. https://healingautoimmune.com/aip-raw-brownie-bites-recipe

Hendon, Louise. Avocado salad. https://healingautoimmune.com/aip-avocado-salad-recipe

Hendon, Louise. Avocado zucchini burgers. https://paleoflourish.com/mini-zucchini-avocado-burgers-recipe

Hendon, Louise. Basil chicken sauté. https://paleoflourish.com/basil-chicken-saute-recipe-paleo-keto-aip

Hendon, Louise. Blueberry coconut popsicles recipe [paleo, dairy-free, aip]. https://paleoflourish.com/blueberry-coconut-popsicles-recipe-paleo-dairy-free

Hendon, Louise. Buddha bowl with sausages. https://healingautoimmune.com/aip-german-sausage-buddha-bowl-recipe

Hendon, Louise. Chicken noodle soup. https://paleoflourish.com/paleo-chicken-noodle-soup-recipe

Hendon, Louise. Chow Mein AIP vegetarian recipe. https://healingautoimmune.com/aip-vegetarian-chow-mein-recipe

Hendon, Louise. Coconut and banana balls. https://paleoflourish.com/coconut-banana-balls-recipe-paleo-gf-dairyfree-nutfree

Hendon, Louise. Cucumber and smoked salmon ham wraps. https://paleoflourish.com/smoked-salmon-lunch-wrap-recipe-paleo-keto

Hendon, Louise. Fish and Leek Saute Recipe [Paleo, AIP, Keto]. https://paleoflourish.com/fish-leek-saute

Hendon, Louise. Fried apricot tuna bites. https://paleoflourish.com/pan-fried-apricot-tuna-salad-bites-recipe

Hendon, Louise. Lamb chops. https://healingautoimmune.com/aip-lamb-chops-recipe

Hendon, Louise. Lemon Brussels sprouts with Salisbury steak. https://healingautoimmune.com/aip-salisbury-steak-lemon-brussels-sprouts-recipe

Hendon, Louise. Lemon tuna salad. https://paleoflourish.com/lemon-black-pepper-tuna-salad-keto-paleo-aip/

Hendon, Louise. Lime chicken and cilantro salad. https://healingautoimmune.com/aip-chicken-lime-cilantro-salad-recipe

Hendon, Louise. Marshmallows. https://healingautoimmune.com/aip-marshmallows-recipe

Hendon, Louise. Mediterranean Tuna salad. https://healingautoimmune.com/aip-mediterranean-tuna-salad

Hendon, Louise. Mussels, mango and carrot hash. https://paleoflourish.com/carrot-mango-mussels-hash-recipe-paleo-aip

Hendon, Louise. Pressure cooker broccoli and beef. https://healingautoimmune.com/aip-pressure-cooker-beef-broccoli-recipe

Hendon, Louise. Pumpkin pie. https://healingautoimmune.com/aip-pumpkin-pie-recipe

Hendon, Louise. Roasted herb pork tenderloin. https://healingautoimmune.com/aip-herb-roasted-pork-tenderloin-recipe

Hendon, Louise. Seafood coconut soup. https://paleoflourish.com/simple-paleo-coconut-seafood-soup-recipe/

Hendon, Louise. Stuffed coconut butter dates. https://paleoflourish.com/coconut-butter-stuffed-dates/

Hendon, Louise. Sweet Potato Carrot Apple Ginger Soup Recipe. https://paleoflourish.com/Sweet-Potato-Carrot-Apple-Ginger-Soup-Recipe

Hendon, Louise. Sweet potato cookies. https://healingautoimmune.com/aip-sweet-potato-cookies-recipe

Hendon, Louise. Waldorf salad. https://healingautoimmune.com/aip-waldorf-salad-recipe

Hendon, Louise. Winter salad. https://healingautoimmune.com/aip-winter-salad

Hendon, Louise. Zoodles and Bolognese. https://healingautoimmune.com/aip-bolognese-zoodles-recipe

Hiromatsu, Yuji, Hiroshi Satoh, and Nobuyuki Amino. "Hashimoto's thyroiditis: history and future outlook." *Hormones (Athens)* 12, no. 1 (2013): 12-8.

Hoover, Michelle. AIP spaghetti squash pizza casserole. https://unboundwellness.com/spaghetti-squash-pizza-casserole/

Hoover, Michelle. AIP unstuffed cabbage roll. https://unboundwellness.com/unstuffed-cabbage-roll/

Hoover, Michelle. Cauliflower oatmeal. https://unboundwellness.com/grain-free-cauliflower-oatmeal/

Hoover, Michelle. Chicken poppers and sausages with a fruit. https://unboundwellness.com/breakfast-sausage-chicken-poppers/

Hoover, Michelle. Ginger cream sauce with egg roll. https://unboundwellness.com/egg-roll-in-a-bowl/

Hoover, Michelle. Paleo Sloppy Joes (AIP). https://unboundwellness.com/paleo-sloppy-joe/

Hoover, Michelle. Skillet Mexican breakfast. https://unboundwellness.com/mexican-breakfast-skillet/

Jay, Kate. Butternut wedges with avocado lime. https://autoimmunewellness.com/spiced-butternut-wedges-with-avocado-lime-mayo/

Jay, Kate. Pumpkin porridge. https://healingfamilyeats.com/aip-pumpkin-porridge-aip/

Jo Teague, Samantha. Creamy artichoke chicken stew (instant pot). https://www.theunskilledcavewoman.com/artichoke-chicken-stew/

Joy, Cassy. Chicken ginger soup. https://fedandfit.com/ginger-chicken-soup/

Kate Jay. Shredded chicken salad (Vietnamese). https://autoimmunewellness.com/vietnamese-shredded-chicken-salad/

Kawicka, Anna, and Bożena Regulska-Ilow. "Metabolic disorders and nutritional status in autoimmune thyroid diseases." *Advances in Hygiene & Experimental Medicine/Postepy Higieny i Medycyny Doswiadczalnej* 69 (2015).

Kong YC, Morris GP, Brown NK, Yan Y, Flynn JC, David CS. Autoimmune thyroiditis: a model uniquely suited to probe regulatory T cell function. J Autoimmun. 2009;33:239-246.

Kristin. Cheese broccoli soup. http://www.wholesomewithin.com/broccoli-cheese-soup/

Laura. Turmeric pork. http://sweet-treats-baking.blogspot.com/2015/12/turmeric-pork-skillet-aip-paleo-whole-30.html

Lemes, de Andrade Isadora, and M. S. Filippovich. "AUTOIMMUNE PROTOCOL: THE USE OF DIET AND LIFESTYLE TO REGULATE THE IMMUNE SYSTEM." pp. 404-406. 2019.

Liontiris, Michael I., and Elias E. Mazokopakis. "A concise review of Hashimoto thyroiditis (HT) and the importance of iodine, selenium, vitamin D and gluten on the autoimmunity and dietary management of HT patients. Points that need more investigation." *Hell J Nucl Med* 20, no. 1 (2017): 51-56.

Marc Ryan, L. A. C. *The Hashimoto's Healing Diet: Anti-inflammatory Strategies for Losing Weight, Boosting Your Thyroid, and Getting Your Energy Back*. Hay House, Inc, 2018.

Marras, Alison. AIP Wild Salmon, Bacon & Pesto Salad. https://foodbymars.com/home/2018/aip-meal-plan/

Marras, Alison. Classic AIP Breakfast Hash. https://foodbymars.com/home/2018/aip-meal-plan/

Marras, Alison. Easy AIP Citrus-Thyme Turkey Breakfast Sausage. https://foodbymars.com/home/2018/aip-meal-plan/

Mori, Kouki, Yoshinori Nakagawa, and Hiroshi Ozaki. "Does the gut microbiota trigger Hashimoto's thyroiditis?." *Discovery medicine* 14, no. 78 (2012): 321-326.

Parvathaneni, Arvin, Daniel Fischman, and Pramil Cheriyath. "Hashimoto's thyroiditis." *A New Look at Hypothyroidism* (2012): 47.

Perillo, Tara. AIP Paleo Instant Pot Beet Fennel Soup Recipe. http://www.paleocajunlady.com/aip-paleo-instant-pot-beet-fennel-soup-recipe/

Raia, Butternut pizzas. https://raiasrecipes.com/2019/05/butternut-pizzas.html

Reaves, Alyssa. Roast chicken with cherries and kale. https://letscreatethesweetlife.com/2018/02/roasted-chicken-with-cherries-and-kale-salad-aip-paleo/

Reaves, Alyssa. Sweet and sour AIP chicken. https://letscreatethesweetlife.com/2018/05/sweet-and-sour-chicken-aip-paleo/

Stauch, Emily. Bratwurst with Brussels sprouts and roasted sweet potatoes. https://flawedyetfunctional.com/food-nutrition/recipe/paleo-recipe-food-nutrition/bratwurst-roasted-veggies/

Schrader, Brent. Chilled Blueberry-Rosemary Soup. https://thatpaleocouple.com/2014/06/25/chilled-blueberry-rosemary-soup-easy-dessert-recipe/

Smith, Joanna. Sweet and Savory Fried Plantains. https://fedandfulfilled.com/sweet-savory-fried-plantains/

Soon, Tan Kar, and Poh Wei Ting. "Journal of Nutritional Disorders & Therapy." (2018).

Spring, Michele. Cassava pancakes. https://thrivingonpaleo.com/aip-cassava-flour-pancakes/

Spring, Michele. Coconut pumpkin pie parfait. https://thrivingonpaleo.com/aip-breakfast-pumpkin-pie-coconut-parfait/

Spring, Michele. Tigernut Chocolate Granola. https://thrivingonpaleo.com/chocolate-tigernut-granola-aip-paleo-vegan-nut-free/

Stevens, Megan. Banana cookies. https://eatbeautiful.net/banana-breakfast-cookies-aip-egg-free-paleo-resistant-starch-collagen-easy-breakfasts-pack-lunches/

Trescott, Mickey. Brussels sprout. https://autoimmunewellness.com/shaved-brussels-sprout-salad/

Trescott, Mickey. Chicken garlic amino kebabs. https://autoimmunewellness.com/garlic-amino-chicken-kebabs/

Trescott, Mickey. Chicken zoodle bowl. https://autoimmunewellness.com/green-chicken-zoodle-bowl/

Trescott, Mickey, and Angie Alt. *The Autoimmune Wellness Handbook: A DIY Guide to Living Well with Chronic Illness.* Rodale, 2016.

Vaidya, Bijay, and Simon HS Pearce. "Management of hypothyroidism in adults." *BmJ* 337 (2008).

Van Tiggelen, Sophie. AIP Breakfast Stack. https://asquirrelinthekitchen.com/85-amazing-aip-breakfasts-a-paleo-autoimmune-protocol-community-cookbook/

Van Tiggelen, Sophie. Bison skillet with broccoli, pomegranate seeds, collard greens, and bacon. https://asquirrelinthekitchen.com/aip-paleo-breakfast-skillet-with-bison-bacon-and-pomegranate-seeds/

Van Tiggelen, Sophie. Cinnamon and vanilla granola. https://asquirrelinthekitchen.com/vanilla-cinnamon-breakfast-granola-paleo-aip-sugar-free-giveaway/

Van Tiggelen, Sophie. Cinnamon, vanilla toasted coconut flakes. https://asquirrelinthekitchen.com/vanilla-cinnamon-toasted-coconut-flakes-paleo-aip-sugar-free/

Van Tiggelen, Sophie. Green smoothie bowl. https://asquirrelinthekitchen.com/energizing-green-breakfast-smoothie-bowl-paleo-aip-coconut-free/

Van Tiggelen, Sophie. Hash casserole with cilantro and butternut squash. https://asquirrelinthekitchen.com/aip-paleo-breakfast-hash-casserole-with-butternut-squash-cilantro/

Van Tiggelen, Sophie. Paleo grain free granola. https://asquirrelinthekitchen.com/paleo-nuttola-grain-free-granola-delicious-gluten-free-breakfast-option/

Van Tiggelen, Sophie. Plum and Apple cake. https://asquirrelinthekitchen.com/apple-plum-breakfast-cake-meal-prep/

Van Tiggelen, Sophie. Thyme and rosemary focaccia bread. https://asquirrelinthekitchen.com/aip-bread/

Van Tiggelen, Sophie. Veggie and protein collagen blend. https://asquirrelinthekitchen.com/vital-proteins-collagen-veggie-blend-review-and-a-recipe/

Whitney. Apple rosemary sausages. https://rootedinhealing.net/2019/10/02/apple-rosemary-breakfast-sausage-aip-whole-30-paleo/

Printed in Great Britain
by Amazon